PULSED YAG LASER SURGERY

DANIÈLE ARON-ROSA, MD
EDITOR

PULSED YAG LASER SURGERY

Dr. Aron-Rosa's work is supported by the
Direction Generale Recherche de Science & Technologie and Electronics Marcel Dassault

Editorial Consultant

Eric M. Baloff
Executive Editor
IOL & OCULAR SURGERY NEWS

6900 Grove Road, Thorofare, New Jersey.

Printed in the United States of America.

ISBN No. 0–943432–03–0
Library of Congress No. 83–060475

This book is dedicated to Edmond De Rothschild and Gabriel Pallez, Director of the Assistance Publique, Paris, not only because they provided all the facilities for my job but mainly for old, warm friendship.

CONTENTS

CONTRIBUTORS

Danièle S. Aron-Rosa, M.D.
Professor of Ophthalmology
Chief of the Eye Clinic
Rothschild Foundation
Trousseau Hospital
Paris, France

Jean-Jacques Aron, M.D.
Professor of Ophthalmology
Chief of the Eye Department of Amboise Paré Hospital
Chief of the Eye Department of the American Hospital
Paris, France

Yvan Atbitbol, M.D.
Chief of the OPD Section
Aron-Rosa Service at the Rothschild Foundation
Trousseau Hospital
Paris, France

R. Birngruber, M.D., Ph.D.
Professor of Ophthalmology
Eye Clinic of the University of Munich
Munich, Germany

K.P. Boergen, M.D.
Assistant in Ophthalmology
Eye Clinic of the University of Munich
Munich, Germany

Cecile M. Boileau-Bonnet, M.D.
Pathologist, Intern of the Hospitals of Paris
Paris, France

Howard C. Cohn, M.D.
Glaucoma Consultant
Chief of the Glaucoma Section
Aron-Rosa Service at the Rothschild Foundation
Trousseau Hospital
Paris, France

B.P. Gabel, M.D.
Professor of Ophthalmology
Eye Clinic of the University of Munich
Munich, Germany

Douglas E. Gaasterland, M.D.
Chief of the Glaucoma Department
Clinical Branch, National Eye Institute
National Institutes of Health
Bethesda, Maryland

Elisabeth Jeanneau, M.D.
Chief of the Clinic of the
Hospitals of Paris
Rothschild Foundation
Trousseau Hospital
Paris, France

Richard D. Keates, M.D.
Professor of Ophthalmology
Eye Institute
Columbus, Ohio

William R. Whalen, M.D.
Ophthalmologist and Glaucoma
Consultant
Littleton, Colorado

Jan G. Worst, M.D.
Gronningen, Holland

H.R. Zink, M.D.
Assistant in Ophthalmology
Eye Clinic of the University
of Munich
Munich, Germany

PREFACE

Il n'est pas nécessaire d'esperer pour entreprendre, ni de réussir pour persévérer.

Guillaume d'Orange.

In that I perform mainly microsurgery, my guidelines have always been to try to be as atraumatic as possible during endocular surgery. Convinced of the superiority of non-invasive methods whenever possible, I tried to build a device capable of cutting the eye without burning or surgically entering it. Since I am a surgeon, and therefore responsible for the best possible care of my patients, I needed a practical, safe, and comfortable device. It seemed obvious to me that this new knife had to be a laser.

After previous experience with argon, ruby, and other lasers, I began working, by random harvest, with pulsed YAG lasers in the early 1970's. Knowing the experimental work of Campbell and Rittler and their attempts in Q-switching ruby lasers, I asked ophthalmic laser manufacturers for a laser that could be pulsed and would be capable of cutting vitreous traction bands without coagulation, thus avoiding the nocive effects of heating the vitreous.

In the beginning, I could not find a company interested in these somewhat unusual concepts, so I tried Q-switched ruby lasers on the rabbit eye. Working in the millisecond range and pulsing so slowly that an enormous amount of millijoules was produced, I exploded a fair number of rabbit eyes without being able to properly perform the experiment. By chance, I encountered Pierre Auger, one of the leaders in post-war nuclear physics. In chatting with him at a dinner party in January 1973, I suddenly understood the significance of *low energy* and *critical power density,* and how important it was to reach *optical breakdown.* He also made clear to me what a plasma meant. In my mind, the three guidelines were settled; what I needed was a low-energy laser at high power density to attain optical breakdown.

I immediately gave up ruby lasers and tried to find a good nanosecond, pulsed YAG laser. Knowing that precise, pulsed lasers were used in wartime industry as range finders for tank cannons, I went to see Serge Dassault who not only provided me with a nanosecond laser, but has since been a supporter of our research laboratory, a friend, and eventually a scientific counselor.

My first YAG was a pocket-sized nanosecond laser provided by the arms industry. This laser worked in the free-running mode, provided an output energy of 40 millijoules, and reached a power density of two megawatts. The pulse duration was 20 nanoseconds and it had the enormous advantage of being a tiny box (40 cm × 40 cm) that attached directly to the top of the slitlamp. A specially treated glass contact lens provided better beam convergence and divergence of the shot without making it too trumpetlike and thus less safe with a longer security distance. At that stage, we already had better results than with the ruby laser but were still far from the degree of precision required.

Chance helped me a second time when, in December 1975, I saw a scientific television show featuring two hematologists (since they then have become Nobel laureates), Dausset and Bessis. They were able to destroy one mitochondrial body inside a blood cell, without exploding the cell, with an ultrarapid, pulsed YAG laser beam. They stressed that the quicker "a train of pulses" (not just one pulse) is sent, the quicker and the more protective the plasma shield will be and the quicker the pulse, the smaller the amount of output energy required to reach optical breakdown in air.

1976 was a year of search and hesitation. The picosecond lasers were only laboratory lasers and I was totally unable (not being a physicist) to build the device myself nor were my usual supporters able to help me. They provided laser rods and pico and nano laboratory instruments, but none of the engineers was able to mount the pico laser. Besides, I had heard that my Swiss neighbor, Fankhauser, who was working with YAG lasers for glaucoma treatment, had given up on the pico YAG, and I did not know what a picolesion on ocular tissue looked like. A few months after that, an unemployed physicist, Jean-Claude Griesemann, a specialist in pulsed lasers, came to see me for two reasons: he knew what I was working on and he wanted me to examine the accidental pico laser lesion he had made on one of his macula. As soon as I saw the perfectly round, limited retinal lesion, without leakage under fluorescein angiography, I knew what I needed and recruited his services. This started the collaboration that brought us to writing this book and to successfully treating more than 7,000 patients.

Which is better: the nano or the pico? In my opinion, both work. The new generation of nanosecond, pulsed lasers is far more precise and safe than its predecessors. Both nano and pico lasers have their own advantages and defects. They are the present lasers and may be either improved or abandoned for better and/or different lasers.

Nano or pico? I will always have a soft spot in my heart for both of them because they permitted me to reach my dream: the non-thermal, precise cutting of intraocular tissues without surgically opening the eye.

Actually, the first person to think of using cold lasers in anterior segment surgery was not me but my husband, Jean Jacques Aron. He sent me capsulotomies from the congenital cataracts he had operated on years before, saying that if the YAG worked safely close to the retina, it was certainly safe and more frequently indicated for posterior capsulotomies, especially behind implants.

Danièle S. Aron-Rosa MD

ACKNOWLEDGEMENTS

I wish to thank Charles Bouquety, who is responsible for the Photography Department, and Raymond Kwort, Mireille Andre, Corine Croq, Pascale Caresmel, Claire de Mangou, and Denise Noirot, who helped greatly.

I am also grateful to Mrs. Jacqueline Delacourt and Pierre Dhermy, the pathologists of the Rothschild Foundation, for their capable assistance.

INTRODUCTION

Pulsed YAG lasers are the latest, but certainly not the last, lasers to be introduced inside the eye as a blade.

Campbell and Rittler (1968) were the first to attempt to cut vitreous traction bands with heavy Q-switched ruby lasers that worked in several-milliseconds duration. Although their knife was explosive and inaccurate, they were 20 years ahead of their time. Since 1968, laser and computer technology has improved so much that radial keratotomy may soon be performed in a few seconds with 100% accuracy using a computerized YAG laser.

Historically, we used lasers with bursts measured in milliseconds, then in nanoseconds, and now in picoseconds. It may not be long before the picosecond laser will be replaced by the phemtosecond laser!

Ophthalmologists are familiar with laser photocoagulation, but most do not have a strong enough background in physics to understand the mechanics of the YAG laser. I remember that when I first presented the picosecond YAG laser in 1979, very few ophthalmologists understood:

1. The difference between continuous and pulsed wave light emission;
2. What a so-called "plasma shield" was;
3. What optical breakdown meant;
4. How you could use a laser without burning tissue;
5. What a nanosecond and a picosecond were;
6. What monomode meant; and
7. What the difference was between active Q-switching and passive Q-switching through a dye (the so-called "mode-locked" laser).

The purpose of this book is to try, using the simplest language possible, to clarify all of these points, so that ophthalmologists who are going to use laser knives will be "in" for the present and prepared for the future in lasers. Hopefully, this book will also inspire new ideas, and, who knows, perhaps its readers will take part in the development of the next generation of ophthalmic lasers.

PULSED YAG LASER SURGERY

Danièle S. Aron-Rosa, M.D.

CHARACTERISTICS OF THE PICOSECOND YAG LASER

1

Characteristics: The picosecond pulsed Neodymium (Nd) YAG laser we built is monomode and mode-locked.*

What does this mean?

Mode-locking means passive Q-switching through a dye. This laser consists of a dye cell which is placed inside the optical resonator between the laser medium and the rear mirror. A saturable absorber (the dye) is used in the dye cell (Fig. 1). A dye used to mode-lock a laser must have a fast recovery time; but dyes with rapid recovery are the least durable.

Nd YAG lasers are mode-locked with Eastman Kodak n° 9740 or 9860 saturable absorbers diluted with 1-2 dichloroethane or chlorobenzene, but 14015 saturable absorber is more stable and durable after dilution.

When the light intensity increases, the absorption coefficient decreases; the more intense the light beam the more transparent the dye becomes (dye bleaching phenomenon) (Fig. 2).

When the dye bleaches suddenly, the laser radiation is allowed to reach the rear mirror (or reflector) and laser oscillation occurs.

What is the mechanism of the bleaching process?

The dye molecules absorb photons and are transferred to an excited state from ground level. When enough molecules are excited, the dye bleaches (which means it has become totally transparent to laser radiation). Up to now, all the dyes that were used with the picosecond YAG laser came from Eastman Kodak. The first were the saturable absorber Q-switch solutions n° 9860 and 9740. To increase the effective life of the dye, we now use the more stable solution n° 14015. To achieve nearly perfect mode-locking, the dye is diluted in either iodoethane, methylsulfoxide, or ethylsulfide.

Temporal and spectral aspects of the output of a dye Q-switched laser depend strongly on the dye relaxation time (the time it takes the dye to return to color). *Mode-locking* means a very short relaxation time. In this case, and only in this case, peak power pulses are obtained in the picosecond range.

The Advantages of Passive Q-Switching and Mode-Locking

The advantages of passive Q-switching and mode-locking are that operation of the laser is simplified, and that pulse output occurs in a narrow waist. This means it is easier to aim at the target tissue, easier to reach optical breakdown with a shorter well-defined spark, and therefore there is more security.

The main disadvantage of the passive Q-switch is that the dye must be changed periodically, although the procedure is quick and simple.

The dye is sensitive to UV light, heat and modifications of the solvents' index of refraction. Five years ago, I had to change the dye every two weeks on an early prototype. Now, the laser may work perfectly mode-locked for at least two to three months without even adding new dye.

To achieve this result (a long-life dye), an UV filter able to reduce dye disintegration was installed and the dye is circulated through a self-enlarged container; the pumping action assuring uniform mixing of the dye. Because of the large volume, the dye concentration remains constant over a long period of time, and fresh dye is exposed to each laser pulse. Temperature, being very important, is permanently monitored. In the newer pico lasers, a dye replenishing feature has been added.

Active Mode-Locking Is Also Possible

Up to this point, I have been addressing passive Q-switching. However, active mode-locking is also possible.

What does this mean?

A phase modulator, placed inside a laser cavity (driven at exactly the frequency separation of the axial mode) can lead to generation of mode-locked pulses: active mode-locking performed on continuous wave pumped lasers is achieved by inserting an electro-optic or

*** The principles of the Nd YAG laser and the basic differences between Q-switching and mode-locking are illustrated in Figures 1-6.**

acousto-optic modulator into the resonator. Both active and passive mode-locking may be used on the same laser.

Active mode-locking works at lower energy levels. Active and passive together offers a higher energy laser.

Mode-Locked or Phase-Locked Laser

In a mode-locked or phase-locked laser, the oscillating modes are in phase. In a *free-running* laser, both longitudinal and transverse modes oscillate simultaneously, with the amplitudes of the different modes being out of phase. Ultrashort pulses in the picosecond range are obtained for solid state lasers only by mode-locking.

Monomode

A monomode state can exist when the divergence of the laser beam is reduced to a minimum. A laser is called monomode when the whole energy is delivered along one axis. If optical breakdown and plasma are not obtained, the focal distance has to be reduced by placing an objective lens on the cornea. A highly convergent contact lens, greater than +45 diopters will give a short focal distance (not exceeding 10 to 20 millimeters) and higher precision for the operator.

Danièle S. Aron-Rosa, M.D.

THE PICOSECOND YAG LASER IN OPHTHALMOLOGY

2

The first prototype YAG laser we built in our laboratory six years ago was a modulated monomode, mode-locked picosecond YAG laser. This device is frequently referred to as the Aron-Rosa laser.

Now, the picosecond laser is stabilized at $\pm 3\%$ crest-to-crest energy. This second-generation laser may be both passive Q-switched through a dye and/or active Q-switched through an electro-optical system that allows the possibility of changing the output energy.

In the prototype, the output energy delivered at each shot ranged from three to seven millijoules in a burst of seven pulses (peaks). Each peak has a 25-picosecond duration. Seven nanoseconds separate one peak from another. The peak energy starts at very low levels for the first pulses, increases until the peak power is reached, then decreases for the last pulses (Fig. 7).

These conditions are mandatory to reach a cumulative and efficient plasma. The interposition of filters improves the ability to graduate the output energy from one to seven millijoules.

The concentration of the low emergent energy in an extremely sharp focus of the beam gives high power density (1.5×10^{12} watt/cm^2): for one millijoule output energy the power density at the focal point is 1×10^{12} watt/cm^2 (Fig. 8).

This concentrated energy, in a very small volume, induces the formation of a shock wave that expands radially from the point of focus disintegrating the target tissue, (Fig. 9) *the laser matter interaction is called optical breakdown.* Optical breakdown occurs when electric fields are strong enough to rip electrons off of atoms, causing ionization of the medium and formation of a plasma. This is similar to the generation of an electric spark during a storm. Optical breakdown leads to the non-linear absorption of the beam in normally transparent tissues. This results in the vaporization of the target tissue at the focal point and the creation of a shock wave that expands radially and disrupts the adjacent tissue, regardless of its site nature and/or color. In the case of the picosecond laser beam pulsed in a train of seven pulses, the optical breakdown is not a point but a linear surface. The size of the spark is $D \sim 0.5$ up to 0.7 mm which, joined to the known diffusion of shock and pressure waves in the vitreous, leads to a harmless shot to the retina of up to 1 to 1.50 mm from the retina. Atoms at the focal point are dissociated into electrons and ions by the electromagnetic field, so creating a plasma cloud, (ionized gas) which is a shield that protects deeper formations such as the retina and is seen clinically as small bubbles. The quicker the plasma shield is created, the better the protection. The quicker the laser pulses, the faster the plasma shield is created. However, the use of a train of pulses permits a cumulative "plasma shield" effect.

The electron density of the ionized gas 10^{21} e/cm^2) makes it reflective at a 1064-nanometers wavelength thus nearly completely blocking the transmission of radiation towards the retina. The shock wave that develops from the energy irradiation zone boundary will be blocked posteriorally by the plasma shield, but will expand frontally towards the more superficial formations (Fig. 10).

Such a process is quite independent of the chemical matter of target, and makes it efficient, regardless of the color or transparency of the tissue to be cut.

No coagulation will be seen. [The pulsed picosecond lasers may be considered cold lasers. It has been calculated that the energy deposit of a millijoule induces a front shock pressure P. At a distance of 0.1 mm $P = 10^7$ mm Hg during 2×10^{-9} seconds. If for the sake of simplicity we considered the eyeball as a sphere of 20 mm diameter, the temperature increase for such a deposit of energy has been calculated not to exceed 2×10^{-3} centigrade, which can be considered not harmful to the eye structures.] A shot focalized on a blood vessel will make it bleed.

The Neodymium (Nd) YAG laser beam is invisible. Therefore, a red helium neon laser beam coincident to the YAG is used for aiming. Operator protection is assured by filters in the eye pieces of the slitlamp, protecting against backward reflection. The maximum irradiation to be received by the operator falls under the ED-50 safety level by a factor of 10^6.

Why I Used Several Pulses

During our preliminary experiments, the

transmitted energy has been measured by a Gentec ED 200 calorimeter. For the usual train of seven pulses of 30 picoseconds each, in a Gaussian envelope, the transmission factor which is inferior to 8%, was found far higher, 20 to 38%, when using a selector of pulses and pulsing only one 30 picoseconds spike at the peak power level; these facts lead us to the conclusion of the importance of the cumulative constitution of the plasma cloud.

Douglas E. Gaasterland, M.D.

FUNDAMENTAL ASPECTS OF LIGHT AND LASERS FOR THE OPHTHALMOLOGIST

3

Introduction

The use of lasers to perform noninvasive ophthalmic surgery has become widespread during the past ten years. In some cases, this has revolutionized surgical technique. Some procedures that previously required invasion of the anterior chamber in the operating room can now be performed noninvasively in an outpatient setting by focused laser light. Ophthalmologists and the public are rapidly accepting these new laser light surgical techniques.

Laser treatment permanently alters target tissue. The ophthalmologist should have an understanding of the interaction between laser light and tissue before using laser surgical techniques. Particularly important is a grasp of the physical concepts related to highly focused light. Small quantities of light are sufficient for eye surgery with lasers; the ophthalmologist should be able to quantify and judge the quality of the light. Similarly, the ophthalmic surgeon must possess an understanding of other instruments used in eye surgery. The purpose of this chapter is to briefly review some fundamental laser concepts and parameters. More extensive and detailed publications are available and should also be consulted.[1]

Physical Properties of Light

All electromagnetic radiation, including light, can be conceptualized as being composed of bundles of energy, which have been called "photons". Photons have both electronic and magnetic properties. In some ways, they behave like waves and, in others, they behave like particles.

The physics of wave motion apply to photons. The velocity of any wave motion is the frequency "ν" of the waves times the wavelength "λ", that is

$$V=(\lambda\nu). \qquad \text{(Eq. 1)}$$

The electromagnetic radiation of the photon is composed of oscillating electric and magnetic fields, and the radiation obeys the frequency-wavelength equation. The velocity of propagation of light is maximal in a vacuum (c_0) and slows in a medium (c). The velocity of light in a vacuum is approximately 3×10^{10} centimeters per second. The wave equation for light is

$$c_0=3\times10^{10}=(\lambda\nu). \qquad \text{(Eq. 2)}$$

The index of refraction "n" is defined as the ratio of the speed of light in a vacuum to the speed of light in the medium that is transmitting light, or

$$n=c_0/c. \qquad \text{(Eq. 3)}$$

Before proceeding with a discussion of the energy in light, several units and definitions are important. These follow:

1. ISAAC NEWTON'S LAW. Force = mass × acceleration;

   $$f=(ma). \qquad \text{(Eq. 4)}$$

2. DYNE. The force to accelerate one gram of mass at a rate of one centimeter per second per second.
3. NEWTON. The force to accelerate one kilogram of mass at a rate of one meter per second per second;

   $$1 \text{ NEWTON}=10^5 \text{ dynes}. \qquad \text{(Eq. 5)}$$

4. WORK. Work is force applied × distance moved.
5. JOULE. One joule is the work of one Newton applied through a distance of one meter. It is a unit of ENERGY.

   $$1 \text{ JOULE}=10^7 \text{ dyne-cm}. \qquad \text{(Eq. 6)}$$

   ERG. One erg is the work of one dyne applied through a distance of one centimeter.
6. POWER. This is how fast energy is produced.
7. WATT. This is the power associated with energy production at a rate of one joule per second.
8. ENERGY DENSITY. This is the energy applied per unit area. Units are joules/cm^2 for lasers.
9. POWER DENSITY. This is the power per unit area. Units are watts/cm^2 for lasers.
10. OPTICAL BREAKDOWN THRESHOLD. This is the power density (or field strength) that causes the onset of "nonlinear" events, for example, ionization or the formation of a gas-filled cavity at the focus of a laser. The optical breakdown threshold is approximately 3×10^{12} watts/cm^2 in air; it is approximately 3×10^{10} watts/cm^2 in water.

Some properties of electromagnetic radiation are more understandable when the radiation is analyzed as photons or discrete bundles of energy. Max Planck (1900) first proposed that the energy in each photon, Q_q, is proportionate to the frequency with which it is vibrating, or

$$Q_q = (h\nu), \qquad \text{(Eq. 7)}$$

where h, the proportionality constant, is Planck's constant. It has been shown that Planck's constant, h, is 6.6×10^{-34} joule-seconds. The quantum theory of Niels Bohr (1911) arose from the consideration of how much energy is in light. It was recognized that the most common sources of electromagnetic radiation with a wavelength of between 10 nanometers and one millimeter were transitions of the electrons of atoms or molecules between a higher energy state (E_1) and the low-energy baseline state (E_0). The quantum theory shows that energy in photons emitted from a high-energy (excited) atom or molecule is equal to the energy that separates the excited and baseline states, and that the energy in the photons occurs in discrete values; thus

$$Q_q = (E_1 - E_0) = (h\nu). \qquad \text{(Eq. 8)}$$

The transition of an electron of a simple, excited atom from the higher energy orbit to the baseline orbit is illustrated (Fig. 11). The photon emitted in this transition has an energy content equal to the difference between the energy states of the two orbits. This determines the frequency of vibration of the photon, since it must obey equation 8 and, hence, its wavelength, since it must obey equation 2.

These considerations allow calculation of the amount of energy present in visible photons. Red photons have a wavelength of approximately 700 nanometers or 7×10^{-7} meters. From the wave equation and the speed of light in a vacuum (equation 2), it is possible to calculate the frequency of oscillation of the photon. The energy is then calculated from Planck's equation (equation 7). It is 2.9×10^{-19} joules/red photon. For green photons, the wavelength is approximately 500 nanometers or 5×10^{-7} meters. Using this, the energy in a single green photon is calculated to be 4×10^{-19} joules. Thus, a single green photon is more energetic than a single red photon. The "electron volt" has been defined as an energy unit equal to 1.602×10^{-19} joules. Therefore, a red photon has an energy of 1.8 electron volts and a green photon has an energy of 2.5 electron volts.

Lasers

General Considerations. "LASER" is an acronym standing for *L*ight *A*mplification by *S*timulated *E*mission of *R*adiation. Light amplification occurs in substances that are able to enter a metastable, higher-energy state when they are exposed to an exciting stimulus. Outer electrons are driven to a high-energy orbit, then spontaneously fall part way to the ground state and enter another, relatively stable orbit. This is illustrated (Fig. 12).

In the metastable, excited state, potential energy is stored as the electron orbits above the ground state. If a photon having the proper electric and magnetic field strengths passes nearby while the medium is in the higher, metastable energy level, the electrons are stimulated to fall to the baseline state and the stored energy is released in the form of a photon that has an identical wavelength and frequency of oscillation as the stimulating photon. Thus, this phenomenon is a stimulated emission of radiation.

Lasers have three basic components, as shown (Fig. 13). The first is the source of *excitation,* which can be electrical, optical, or thermal energy. The second component is the laser *medium,* which can be either solid, liquid, or gas. The third component is the *cavity,* which includes the medium and is bounded by mirrors. The mirror at the rear of the cavity is usually highly (or nearly totally) reflective; the mirror at the front of the cavity is usually only partially reflective. This mirror allows a part of the incident light to escape the cavity and is therefore the output mirror.

Three steps occur in the event of lasing. First, the source of excitation causes a population inversion in the medium. The excitation energy causes a majority of the available electrons of the medium to move to a metastable, high-energy state. Second, some of the excited electrons drop spontaneously to the base level. There is an associated release of photons that interact with electrons of other excited atoms without being absorbed. Since the photons have the proper electromagnetic field, they stimulate a chain reaction of transitions. The photons have the same wavelength, phase, and direction. Third, the mirrors of the cavity propagate the chain reaction by creating a resonating movement of photons back and forth between the front and rear mirrors. Since the front mirror is only partially reflective, some of the photons escape the cavity and propagate away from the laser.

Laser light has several general characteristics. The *brightness* of laser output exceeds all known man-made and natural light sources in terms of power density (energy per second per unit area). Laser light has *low divergence*. Light rays leaving the laser cavity are nearly parallel. The total included angle between the outermost rays of the bundle is usually measured in terms of approximately one milliradian. One milliradian is approximately 0.05 degrees. The focal spot of collimated laser light on the human retina (approximately 16 micrometers) is about one-tenth the diameter of the image of the sun on the retina.

The light output of a laser is *monochromatic*; one or more specific wavelengths is characteristic of each type of laser medium. A summary of wavelengths that are characteristic for ophthalmic lasers is found in Table I. The light emitted from lasers is *coherent*. This means that the oscillations of the waves of electromagnetic radiation in laser light occur simultaneously in both time and space. The peaks are separated by the wavelength of the light (Fig. 14). The phenomenon of *laser speckle* is characteristic. This is the striking granular appearance that can be seen in reflected laser light. It occurs due to reinforcement and interference when the laser light reflects from a comparatively rough surface. The speckle pattern appears to move as the viewer moves because the reinforcement and interference occur in different locations. Another characteristic of laser radiation is its *mode structure*. Oscillations that occur in the cavity with a component perpendicular to the centerline cause an off-center buildup of energy in the output beam. As a result, the distribution of energy deviates from the Gaussian distribution found in laser beams that do not have a perpendicular component to the oscillations. These *transverse modes* are very important in lasers that might be used for ophthalmic applications because they increase the minimum focal spot diameter. In addition to the transverse modes, there can be more than one harmonic oscillation along the cavity length. This leads to *longitudinal modes* of oscillation. As a consequence, there is a slight loss of sharpness of the output wavelength and frequency. The longitudinal modes fall off very sharply from around the central, characteristic wavelength of the laser.

TABLE I

Characteristic wavelengths of lasers used for ocular treatment

Laser Medium	Wavelength (nm)	Color
Argon	488.0	Blue
	514.5	Green
Nd-YAG (2nd harmonic)	532.0	Green
Helium-neon	632.0	Orange-red
Krypton	647.0	Red
Ruby	694.0	Red
Nd-YAG (1st harmonic)	1064.0	Infrared
Erbium-YLF	1228.0	Infrared
Carbon dioxide	10,600.0	Infrared

Continuous-Wave Lasers. In general, lasers are classified in two categories—those that are continuously operating, called "continuous-wave" lasers, and those that are pulsed. Continuous-wave lasers are constant in output. They have an efficiency of one to two percent in conversion of input energy to output energy. Continuous lasers have been widely used in ophthalmology for coagulation or burning of target tissue. The rate of production of energy by these lasers is comparatively slow. An argon laser operating at one watt delivers 0.1 joule, or 100 millijoules, in 0.1 second. The lasing media of the continuous-wave lasers that have been in use in ophthalmology include argon, krypton, carbon dioxide, neodymium-glass, and neodymium-YAG (yittrium-aluminum-garnet).

Pulsed Lasers. Pulsed lasers differ from continuous-wave in that the excitation of pulsed lasers is on for only a brief time. Excitation is typically derived from the light of a flashlamp or another laser, or from a short application of electric energy. The lasing media in pulsed lasers can be liquid, crystalline, or gas. Crystalline-pulsed lasers have been widely used for many years. Examples are lasers in which the lasing medium is a ruby crystal, a neodymium-glass crystal, or a neodymium-YAG crystal. In recent years, pulsed neodymium-YAG lasers have developed a high degree of reliability and reproducibility of output. This contributes to their popularity for ophthalmic application.

For ten years, since the pioneering work of Krasnov,[2,3] high-powered, pulsed laser systems have been in ophthalmic use. These lasers have ultrashort pulses due to being assembled with a shutter-like device between the mirrors of the laser cavity. The shutter "spoils" the continuity of the cavity during the initial milliseconds after excitation is applied to the crystalline medium. Since the cavity cannot resonate (the shutter blocks it), a large amount of potential energy accumulates in the metastable orbits of the medium. When the shutter device is opened, the laser cavity empties itself of its stored energy in a very short interval. The duration is measured either in nanoseconds or picoseconds. Conventional pulsed lasers do not have a shutter in the cavity but have a multiple-pulse output, with the duration of each pulse measured in microseconds. A very high power is present in the output beam of pulsed lasers with a shutter in the cavity because the photons are packed into a pulse of very short duration.

Types of Pulsed-Laser Shutters and Effects on Function. Two types of shutter devices are used in ophthalmic-pulsed laser systems. The first is a shutter that results in *mode-locking.* This is usually a passive device and consists of a cell containing a solution of a specific dye. The photosensitive dye is in a thin layer in the cell and is located in the laser cavity adjacent to the back reflector. When the laser medium is excited, photons that are released start to bleach the dye. When sufficient bleaching occurs, the pathway between the mirrors of the laser cavity is opened to photons and the light amplification process occurs. An intrinsic property of the dye is that its recovery time after bleaching is very fast, typically four to five picoseconds. The result of interaction of the dye cell with the photons is a single pulse of light with a duration measured in picoseconds. Activity in the cavity then ceases until some of the photons have made the round trip of the laser cavity and again encounter the dye cell. Bleaching again occurs and another pulse is generated. In this way, a chain of pulses is created. The time separating any two pulses in the chain is that for photons to travel the length of the laser cavity and back. Mode-locked lasers have a long cavity, usually longer than one meter. Since the dye cell is located at the end of the cavity next to the back reflector, there is either reinforcement or cancellation of various harmonic oscillation modes within the cavity; this is the origin of the phase- or mode-locking.

The second type shutter is the Q-switch. For most modern lasers, this is an electro-optic device. This polarizing shutter is usually located within the laser cavity at a distance from the reflectors. The plane of polarization of a crystal in the shutter is normally perpendicular to the plane of polarization of the light coming out of the medium. A short duration voltage pulse from the laser electric system causes the plane of polarization of the crystal in the shutter to rotate 90 degrees. As a result, the polarized laser light can pass the shutter and oscillation can occur in the cavity. The cavity of Q-switched lasers is usually less than half a meter in length and can be as short as eight to ten centimeters. The Q-switch is a slow shutter compared to the dye cell used for mode-locked lasers. As a consequence, the pulse of laser light generated by an electro-optic Q-switch is typically 10 to 30 nanoseconds in duration. A single pulse from a mode-locked laser has a duration of 30 to 100 picoseconds. Electro-optic Q-switches are reliable and require little maintenance. They often function for many thousands of cycles without failure. The passive dye cell is similarly reliable, but requires that the photosensitive dye be replaced periodically.

Ophthalmic Pulsed Laser Systems. The modern pulsed laser systems, both Q-switched and mode-locked, being used in ophthalmic systems are usually selected to operate in the fundamental transverse excitation mode

(TEM_{00}). Most have a near-Gaussian distribution of energy in the physical cross section of the laser beam. As a result, the focal spot diameter of these lasers is as small as is physically possible. When pulsed lasers are combined with ophthalmic delivery systems, the focal spot diameter is typically near 50 micrometers. In contrast, early, Q-switched, ophthalmic, ruby laser systems were multimodal. The output was non-Gaussian, and the smallest spot diameter for these systems often exceeded 200 micrometers.

Empirical studies have shown that both Q-switched and mode-locked neodymium-YAG laser pulses, with energy content from one to five millijoules, are sufficiently energetic to cause punctures within anterior ocular tissue at the focus. In the case of the mode-locked laser, energy is delivered in a train of six to ten small pulses. Each pulse is separated by five to six nanoseconds. Therefore, the total duration of the mode-locked train is about 50 nanoseconds.

In ophthalmic systems, the energy content of neodymium-YAG pulses is adjustable. Filters can be placed in the path of the beam just outside the cavity of both Q-switched and mode-locked lasers. The filters absorb a part of the energy. In addition, the voltage setting to charge the capacitors for the flashlamp of Q-switched lasers can be adjusted up or down. This changes the energy content of the Q-switched pulse. Examples of characteristic output parameters for Q-switched and mode-locked neodymium-YAG lasers are found in Table II. The average power for Q-switched lasers is characteristically a million watts; for mode-locked lasers, it is an order of magnitude higher for any one of the pulses comprising the pulse train. The energy density, from the focused pulse of either the Q-switched or mode-locked neodymium-YAG systems, is characteristically anywhere from ten to more than 100 J/cm^2 when the laser is operating in the TEM_{00} mode and the entire pulse train from the mode-locked laser system is considered. The power density obtained from focused, Q-switched, neodymium-YAG laser pulses is on the order of 10^{10} $watts/cm^2$; the power density for any one of the pulses of the pulse train from a mode-locked system is an order of magnitude larger than the Q-switched power density. The explanation is that the duration of the single mode-locked pulse is 500 to 1000 times shorter than the Q-switched pulse, while the energy content of the single mode-locked pulse is approximately ten times less.

TABLE II

Typical characteristics of focused Q-switched and mode-locked TEM_{00} neodymium-YAG laser applications from ophthalmic systems

	Q-switched	Mode-locked
Focal spot diameter (micrometers)	60	60
Number pulses	1	7
Duration each pulse (seconds)	10×10^{-9}	25×10^{-12}
Energy/application (millijoules)	6	5
Energy/pulse (millijoules)	6	0.7
Energy density (joules/cm^2)	212	25
Power/pulse (megawatts)	0.6	28
Power density (watt/msc^2)	2×10^{10}	99×10^{10}

The high energy and power density in the output from focused, pulsed lasers impose design constraints on ophthalmic, pulsed-laser delivery systems. When laser light from a pulsed laser is focused upon a small area, it may damage the surface of optical elements. If the pulse of light is brought to a focus within the delivery system before it gets to the eye, it is likely that optical breakdown will occur at the focal point. This may reduce the effectiveness of the laser pulse when it gets to the tissue target. Currently available fiber optic bundles cannot be used to deliver high-power, pulsed laser light from the cavity to the ophthalmic microscope because internal focusing in fiber optic bundles would damage the glass fibers. As a result, the laser cavity must be adjacent to the ophthalmic microscope or connected to it by an articulated arm system that contains specially coated, damage-resistant mirrors. For anterior segment treatment with pulsed lasers, it is important to expand the collimated laser beam to a diameter of four to five centimeters before it is focused. This results in a large angle of convergence between the objective lens of the system and the focal point, and a large angle of divergence beyond the focal point. The former tends to protect the cornea and the latter tends to protect the retina during treatment of pupillary membranes. The four-centimeter diameter with a 100-millimeter focal length objective result in a cone angle, the total angle of convergence of the laser beam, close to 20 degrees. Use of plastic examining lenses for pulsed laser treatment and application of laser pulses to tissue targets adjacent to plastic intraocular lenses is possible because of the large cone angle. Damage of the plastic lens is less likely because the laser pulse is of lower energy density at the location of the plastic substrate.

High-powered, pulsed, neodymium-YAG laser systems are within the Class IV category of the Bureau of Radiological Health of the U.S. Department of Health and Human Services.[4] The regulations for radiation control require that Class IV lasers be equipped to measure the energy in each pulse. Other useful features are a pulse counter and a footswitch for activating the system. Another useful feature is a visible aiming beam to indicate the location of the focus of the laser system. The pulsed neodymium-YAG output is in the near-infrared spectral region and, therefore, invisible. Also, since the pulsed laser is only activated momentarily, the focus cannot be identified when it is not active. The beam of a helium-neon laser (wavelength 632 nanometers) is used in most neodymium-YAG, pulsed, ophthalmic laser systems to localize the focal point. The aiming beam uses the same final focusing optics as the infrared beam. Before it comes to the objective lens of the system, the aiming beam is made to diverge slightly so that its focal point will coincide with that of the longer wavelength infrared light.

Effects of Lasers on Ocular Tissue and Plastic Lenses. Eight parameters determine the effect of laser radiation on tissue. These are the following:

1. *Wavelength* of the source
2. *Absorbance* or *transmittance* of the tissue
3. *Image area* or *diameter* at the target
4. *Duration* of the exposure
5. *Energy* delivered to the target
6. *Power* delivered to the target
7. *Energy density* of the radiation at the target site
8. *Power density* of the radiation at the target site

Examples taken from studies of threshold chorioretinal laser lesions help to clarify the importance of the parameters. Damage from exposure of chorioretinal tissue to laser applications of one millisecond or longer is due to thermal injury (burning) and requires ten to fifty joules/cm^2. The energy density required to cause a threshold lesion is higher when the applications have a longer duration. With these long exposures, tissue is damaged by denaturation of protein, with inactivation of enzymes. When pulses of light of very short duration, measured in microseconds or shorter, are applied to chorioretinal tissue, the exposure ends before there is much flow of heat away from the target site. As a result, the threshold lesion is confined to the target site and a small, adjacent area is affected by nonthermal processes. Bleeding commonly follows this type of treatment because the tissue is punctured by the focused pulse without coagulation of the edges of the wound. The threshold chorioretinal lesion from a pulse of microsecond duration occurs with an energy density of about 0.5 joules/cm^2.

For Q-switched pulses with durations of 20 to 50 nanoseconds, the energy density required for the threshold lesion is higher, being approximately one joule/cm^2. The explanation for the larger threshold that occurs with tissue damage from shorter pulses is that superheating and other events in the tissue at the target site absorb extra energy. The temperature within the target site may exceed 200,000 degrees. Pigment granules can be heated to more than 1000 degrees centigrade. Energy is absorbed by the generation of photoacoustic (mechanical) and ionization (chemical) events caused by the high energy density of the short focused pulse. When pulsed laser energy above the threshold is delivered to the chorioretinal tissue, more extensive alteration occurs, including the formation of gas bubbles.

Most ophthalmic laser systems can cause energy densities and power densities that exceed the threshold for nonlinear interactions. When this occurs, the laser system has packed photons together with such density that the local electric field strength induces ionization in the target molecules. The duration of the event is short; therefore, heat does not diffuse to surrounding regions. Although a very high temperature is generated at the focal point, there is negligible effect upon the temperature of the whole eye because the total amount of energy delivered to the eye is modest. The high energy density at the focal point, however, is sufficient to create a microexplosion. This occurs in the absence of absorption of energy by the target and, indeed, can happen in transparent targets. The threshold for optical breakdown, with microexplosions, in water is about 3×10^{10} watts/cm^2 and in air is about 3×10^{12} watts/cm^2. Reaching or exceeding the threshold is associated with creation of a visible, white light spark in the focal area. Such nonlinear effects are seen after application of either Q-switched or mode-locked, neodymium-YAG, infrared light pulses to the eye. Some investigators have indicated that the sparking associated with nonlinear events during ocular treatment creates a barrier that is sufficient to protect the retina at a distance behind the focal point. There is no study in the ophthalmic literature to substantiate this possibility.

For Q-switched and mode-locked laser pulses, the damage threshold for membranes in the eye and for plastic intraocular lenses appears to be more related to the energy density than the power density at the focal point.[5] The threshold for damage of plastic intraocular lenses is about six joules/cm^2 for single mode-locked pulses at 1064 nanometers and is 15 joules/cm^2 for single Q-switched pulses at 1064 nanometers. The corresponding power densities are 380 gigawatts/cm^2 for the mode-locked pulses and about one gigawatt/cm^2 for the Q-switched pulses. The threshold for damage of pupillary membranes inside the human eye is similar to that for plastic intraocular lenses. When pupillary membranes are treated with pulsed lasers, it appears that one of the most important parameters for protection of the intraocular lens is the large cone angle used in the design of modern, ophthalmic, pulsed laser systems. The large cone angle results in a lower energy density in the intraocular lens because it is located in front of the focal point on the membrane. Obviously, precise aiming is important. A pulse delivered with a focus slightly anterior to the membrane will be sufficiently intense to cause focal damage to an intraocular lens at that location. The damage threshold for glass substrates, also in air, is two to ten or more times higher than the threshold for damage of plastic intraocular lenses.[6, 7]

References

1. Sliney, D, Wolbarsht, M: Safety with Lasers and Other Optical Sources. A Comprehensive Handbook. New York, Plenum Press, 1980.
2. Krasnov, MM: Laseropuncture of the anterior chamber angle in glaucoma. Am. J. Ophthalmol. 75:674–678, 1973.
3. Krasnov, M: Laser-phakopuncture in the treatment of soft cataracts. Brit. J. Ophthalmol. 59: 96–98, 1975.
4. U.S. Department of Health, Education and Welfare. Regulations for the Administration and Enforcement of The Radiation Control Health and Safety Act of 1968. HEW Publication (FDA) 79–8035. September, 1978. pp. 50–64.
5. Davi, SK, Gaasterland, DE, Liesegang, G: Pulsed laser damage thresholds of membranes and IOLs. Invest. Ophthalmol. Vis. Sci. 24: (abstract, in press), 1983.
6. Boling, NL, Crisp, MD, Dube, G: Laser induced surface damage. Applied Optics. 12:650–660, 1973.
7. Bliss, ES, Milam, D, Bradbury, RA: Dielectric mirror damage by laser radiation over a range of pulse durations and beam radii. Applied Optics. 12:677–689, 1973.

Danièle S. Aron-Rosa, M.D.
Cecile M. Boileau-Bonnet, M.D.
Jan G. Worst, M.D.

THE PICOSECOND, MONOMODE, MODE-LOCKED, LASER-INDUCED LESIONS AND SIDE EFFECTS: PATHOLOGY

4

It was the pathology of the picosecond, monomode, mode-locked, laser-induced lesions and side effects that helped us to understand first, that the *shock wave* was the main purveyor of tissue destruction; second, that you must use the laser properly in order to achieve satisfactory results. Distorting the laser beam will result in distorted pathology; and third, it was through pathology that we learned what the security distance was.

Similar lesions are produced by the picosecond monomode stabilized YAG laser no matter what tissue is involved. The main features of these lesions may be described as follows:

Central cavitations and shrinkage (vitrification) at burst site with very little extension behind the burst site. This is a safety factor for deeper tissues and is due to the narrow waist of the picobeam and to the cumulative effect of the very rapidly induced plasma screen. There is always superficial and radial extension of the shock waves, yet, with all beam positions, this never exceeds 0.5 mm in depth and 300 microns in width. The walls of the canal describing the concentration of the laser beam are smooth, regular, and far more limited than with a nano at the same power density level.

Compared to the nanosecond burst, the pico induced lesion is smaller and more perfectly limited without a transition zone between destroyed and normal cells. It is accompanied by a limited, transient, surrounding swelling without cellular modification and is only seen at very high power densities. The extension of the swelling never exceeds one-fifth of the destroyed tissue. In both animal experiments and clinical experience, no retinal damage was produced unless the beam was focused to within 1.0 to 0.5 mm of the retina. Bleeding had occurred when a blood vessel was hit by the shock wave. But all bleeding was transient and no frank vessel perforation had been observed. The healing of a pico laser-induced lesion is that of a cut and not of a burn, and the lesion was never seen to be evolutive in any tissue.

When Focused in Coaxial Position

The induced destruction, which is not a focal point but a focal line, is almost perfectly circular as all of the energy is being concentrated on one, unique, 50-micron spot. The anterior extension of the shock wave never exceeds a quarter of a millimeter and there is only one lesion located at the focal point. The length of the optical breakdown with the picosecond laser is 0.6 mm to 0.7 mm, which permits a riskless shot at 1.0 to 1.5 mm distance from the retina (ATLAS Figs. A-D).

When Focused in Lateral Position

When the laser beam is aimed from a lateral position, the shot will be oblique and will become a focal line.

The laser beam is distorted by an oblique astigmatism creating two focal zones perpendicular to one another and, consequently, two optical breakdowns occur. In some cases, a linear fracture may be seen running anteriorly from the posterior break according to the nature of the tissue (ATLAS Figs. A-D).

Experimental Shots on the Cornea

Transmission electron microscope studies of YAG laser lesions on the rabbit corneal epithelium are consistent with the laser's theoretical mode of action. Cellular destruction is caused by bursting and not by burning. The borders of the lesion are sharp compared to adjacent, unaffected tissue. The basal layer is respected and there is little reactional edema to the shot area (ATLAS Figs. E-O).

When the laser beam is focused on the corneal epithelium at the cornea-air interface, a shock wave "click" sound is audible. In the coaxial position, the damage induced by a single burst is not consistent. The unique lesion is 60 microns wide and does not involve the stroma. Focusing on the corneal surface with the laser beam in the lateral position produces an oval-shaped lesion.

When the laser beam is focused on the corneal endothelium in the coaxial position

(ATLAS Figs. P-X), the lesion is round, circular, 150 to 250 microns wide, and well limited. Anterior extension of the shock wave is less than 0.25 mm at three millijoules energy output and no stromal swelling is noticed. With energy greater than five millijoules, the surrounding stroma is swollen. However (cf supra), the swollen cells are normal in shape and the ring of swelling will never be larger than 25 microns in width. No lesion of the corneal stroma or epithelium was ever found in or out of the axis of the shot, whatever the power density in the coaxial position (ATLAS Figs. P-X).

When the laser beam is directed from a lateral position, the more lateral the beam, the more ovale and large the endothelium destruction. For one burst, two areas of destruction occur, one at the endothelial level and a second one located on the corneal epithelium at the site of laser beam entrance. A linear fracture appears when high power densities are reached. The longest fracture ever observed is 0.46 millimeters.

Following the laws of beam distortions and astigmatism, the two destructions will occur 90° apart. In dealing with posterior capsulotomy in pseudo-phakic patients, one must be conscious of the fact that a high corneal astigmatism (superior to five diopters) induces a beam distortion even when the beam is aimed in the coaxial position.

YAG Picosecond-Induced Lesions of the Lens

In rabbits, when the focus is coaxial and the burst is focalized deep enough under the anterior capsule layer, the capsule remains intact. The lesion looks like a canal that perforates the entire cortex and does not involve the lens's nucleus. The lesion is round, circular, 80 to 100 microns wide, from 0.3 to 0.7 mm long, and the walls of the canal are perfectly smooth. There is no transition zone between the destroyed canal and the normal, surrounding fibers when the eye is removed immediately after treatment. Several hours later, dissociation of the normal fibers' arrangement becomes visible. At the site of the focal burst, there is a "crater" with shrinkage of the destroyed tissue comparable to that described for the corneal lesion (ATLAS Figs. Y-TT).

When the laser beam is directed from a lateral position the canal is more oblique, longer, and less regular than when in the coaxial position. The nearer to the site of the burst, the smoother the walls of the canal. Opposite the focal point, the lens's fibers look as if they were just repelled by the shock wave, not destroyed or shrunken. In general, when compared, by scanning electron microscopy, to the regular stacking of normal cortical fibers, the lens's fibers after a laser shot have the following characteristics:

In the Immediate Vicinity of the Destroyed Canal:

- The fibers have lost their usual, regular pattern and
- Cortical fibers appear emptied of their contents like an empty honeycomb. Subcapsular epithelium globules are swollen and spread around the borders of the lesion.

Further Away:

- The cortical fibers look swollen, still regular in their structure and shape, and are slightly disociated from each other with a fine exudate covering them all.

When the Burst is Focused on the Anterior Lens Capsule:

- Blow-out of the anterior capsule is visible, together with dissociation and detachment of the cortical fibers;
- The capsule is widely exploded by one shot, whatever the energy output; and
- The lesion has irregularly shredded limits and the capsule borders are lacelike. The shrinkage of the borders of the destroyed capsule results in a far wider hole than the lesion in the lens or on the cornea (extension of the hole results from retraction of the tensed capsule). The capsule is detached from the underlying cortex, whose fibers appear swollen and dissociated. Many cortex epithelium globules are spread through the capsular cleft.

The main lesions: splitting and tearing of the capsule, dissociation, and swelling of the cortical fibers will be more evident if the eye is removed several hours after laser treatment. The capsular opening may facilitate the ECCE procedure. The picosecond laser is too weak to perform rapid and efficient phako-fragmentation, to allow aspiration of the nucleus through less than a two millimeter opening.

This was also reproduced on a human eye in which the anterior capsule was opened 18 hours prior to enucleation. Aside from the capsule opening, swelling of the cortex, and spreading of the epithelium cortex globules, it was evident that, whatever the emergent energy (three to seven millijoules), neither the nucleus nor the posterior cortex or capsule was perforated with one laser shot and no laser-induced lesion was found on the retina.

The picosecond laser-induced lesions on the normal iris are hardly visible whether the beam is coaxial or not. The soft iris rippled under the shock, and we were able to properly perforate a normal iris with the pico YAG-pulsed laser only when a strongly convergent contact lens was used (ATLAS Fig. UU).

The picolaser, monomode-induced lesion on the human trabecular meshwork demonstrated the creation of a regular, open canal, establishing communication with the Shlemm's canal. Most of the anterior trabecular fibers are frayed by the laser burst and the laser shot does not induce swelling of the surrounding meshwork fibers.

Retina

Of the experimental human retinal shots, pathological examination at two to seven days after only one laser shot showed:

At three to four millijoules output energy, a clearly limited tissue disruption with no transition zone between normal and destroyed tissue, no perforation, no hemorrhage on the retina, and no swelling of the normally shaped border cells could be seen on the eye, which was enucleated on the sixth day. The internal limiting membrane of the vitreous was seen undulated but not ruptured. No retinal swelling or detachment was observed on the eye enucleated on the seventh day. The healing was seen to be that of a cut and not of a burn, without any adhesion between the retina and the external layers, and no extensive necrosis had been picolaser-induced (ATLAS Figs. VV, WW).

At five to seven millijoules output energy, the retina was perforated, hemorrhages spread into the vitreous, and the internal limiting membrane was ruptured. Exudation was present under the retina and still present at the fourth day. Choroid and sclera remained normal. No extensive or limited necrosis of the retina did appear. Fluorescein angiography, performed every day from the first day to the enucleation day (fourth-seventh), showed a clearly limited lesion without retinal edema or vascular leakage. A laser shot was produced by an unattached laboratory pico YAG laser. The energy output was above 12 millijoules.

The patient's vision remained 20/60 and, in seven years follow-up, retinal detachment never occurred. Fluorescein angiography showed a limited fenestration on a deeper layer of the retina without CME or leakage. When focusing the laser at 1½ diopters (0.5 mm from the retina) at 3.5 millijoules, no lesion will appear. At over four millijoules, swelling and undulation of the retina or even perforation will occur. These facts clearly show that 1.5 mm is the top security distance from the retina, as proven by theory. It is also clear that blood vessels and their vicinity must be avoided as long as there is no way to coagulate blood vessels with the pico laser. Therefore, YAG-pulsed lasers have been, up to now, contraindicated for diabetic retinal proliferation treatment.

Danièle S. Aron-Rosa, M.D.

THE PICOSECOND YAG LASER IN CATARACT SURGERY

5

The YAG laser has greatly improved implantation surgery. The laser easily performs a posterior capsulotomy and avoids the risks involved in needling the posterior capsule and the ensuing risks of infection; the laser avoids dislocation and the difficulties of cutting a resistant membrane, as well.

How to Use a Pulsed YAG Laser

Currently available pulsed YAG lasers have the laser delivery, either through the slit lamp light source or through the ocular pieces. With either system, delivery can be made coaxial (perpendicular to the target) as is done with argon laser photocoagulators.

Results of recent pathology studies show that an important factor in producing the desired optical breakdown and shock wave is having the incident laser beam perpendicular to the central cornea, i.e. coaxial to the pupillary axis. This means that the part of the slit lamp containing the laser must be in the coaxial position. Keeping both parts coaxial fulfills this requirement, although if an annoying light reflection results, the non-laser part may be moved slightly off axis. When the laser is in lateral position, the beam is distorted, the focal point becomes a focal line, and is astigmatized. Two optical breakdowns occur (not only in water, but even in air): one is anterior and of a very small diameter (about 50 microns) and the second one, deeper, larger (150 microns), and perpendicular to the previous one, is located on an oblique line.

In between the two breakdowns, according to the tissue consistency, occasionally a fine, linear fracture of the tissue may occur. The more oblique the beam, the farther one breakdown is from the other. Maximum distance between two breakdowns with a picosecond beam was 0.5 mm for five to seven millijoules of output energy. From three to four millijoules, no fractures have been observed along the oblique beam and, at three millijoules, the superficial breakdown gave a minimal destruction of 50 microns in diameter and 10 microns in thickness (four cell layers).

An important concept to grasp is that of the security distance.

Security distance may be defined as the length of the spark (0.5 up to 0.7 mm) added to the diffusion ring of both pressure and elastic waves, which may vary according to the consistency of the disrupted tissue. In the coaxial position, the security distance to be respected is 0.008 mm posteriorly (which is deeper) and 0.25 mm anteriorly (which is more superficial). In the lateral position, at thirty degrees from the primary position, the security distance (between 0.4 to 0.75 mm) is much longer due to the beam distortion and production of both double, linear, optical breakdowns. For maximum security, we advise keeping a safe distance of 1.5 mm from the retina.

YAG treatment is not painful. However, when tissues such as the corneal epithelium and iris are treated, the patient may complain of a slight, very brief shock (minor discomfort).

Preparation of the Patient. Both nano and pico lasers are used on an outpatient basis, and no local anesthesia is used unless a three-mirror Goldmann lens or convergent +20 D to +60 D lens is required to reach deeper formations such as vitreous traction bands, to fix an unsteady eye, and/or to reshape the laser beam when the laser is used laterally instead of coaxially. Lateral delivery is not recommended, especially for posterior capsulotomy behind the IOL. Retrobulbar anesthesia, in our experience, is only exceptionally required in case of significant nystagmus.

Conditions for Good Laser Delivery. The following conditions are essential to perform efficient laser treatment: clear media to the target tissues and the presence of at least a shallow anterior chamber are mandatory. A hazy cornea will absorb and diffract light energy, making precise surgery nearly impossible.

In case of very low endothelial cell counts with slight corneal edema, irrigation of the cornea during the laser session is of great help. Methylcellulose solutions are used systematically in patients with dry corneas since a dry cornea will cause diffraction of the laser beam.

Highly vascularized tissue must not be cut with the pulsed YAG unless primarily coagulated by a continuous YAG or argon laser. Up to now, we find argon laser coagulation to be more efficient.

Indications

Opacities in the corneal surface have the potential of blocking low-power Nd YAG irradiation. The elasticity of the cornea results in the transmission of the elastic wave anteriorly from the target point, which may create a second more superficial lesion. Although it may be possible to make corneal incisions with a pulsed YAG, both present mountage and power levels are absolutely inadequate to perform radial keratotomy or limbal keratotomy; it takes too long, comparatively, to effectively produce a practical incision at this time.

Laser treatment with the YAG laser of some surface lesions such as ulcers is possible instead of curettage, and destruction of stromal microabscesses has been already attempted in a few patients by focusing the laser beam on minute spots. However, one must consider the possibility of dispersing and aggravating the problem instead of the desired destruction of infectious lesions.

Another clinical application, which demonstrates the nonthermal effect of the laser, is the cutting of sutures after cataract extraction or keratoplasty.

One more clinical application is the possibility of cutting the prolene loops of an IOL if the IOL is to be removed. The inserted lens must be steadied; otherwise the lens will move in front of the shock wave and its disruption may require over one hundred shots.

From our experience with the monomode, mode-locked laser, at 4.5 millijoules, the section of a 0.2-mm prolene loop on a fixated lens requires between 40 to 50 shots. This was done in two cases prior to IOL removal and resulted in highly successful surgery.

Anterior Capsulotomy and the Lens's Fragmentation

Anterior capsulotomy may be readily done by pulsed YAG lasers. Making a linear series of pulses in the anterior capsule and the cortex a few hours or a day prior to surgery makes the removal of the capsule easier at surgery and removal is accomplished in one piece, and without traction on the zonules. It allows hydration of the lens, which makes extracapsular extraction of the lens easier and has proven to prevent endothelial cell loss at surgery by avoiding one more manipulation in the anterior chamber. In our experience of more than 2,000 ECCE's, the average endothelial cell loss was 7 ± 5% compared to 18 ± 5% when the capsule was not laser-opened before. It shortens the time of usage of mechanical irrigation/aspiration systems, making it easier. The accidental preoperative breaking of the posterior capsule becomes unlikely as long as the cortex detaches spontaneously (Figs. 15, 16).

Problems arise, however, if one performs the anterior capsulotomy too soon. High intraocular pressure or anaphylactic or immune response to the cortical material may occur if too many days elapse before surgery or if the patient was previously sensitized to the lens material. It is recommended not to open the capsule more than one to three hours before surgery when the lens is soft and the cataract is hypermature, and not to open it at all in case of glaucoma.

The criticism has been made that it may be more difficult to obtain pupillary dilatation if an anterior capsulotomy is performed a day prior to surgery.

In our experience, unless accidental shots have been made on the iris (which may occur in shooting laterally and not coaxially), the pupillary dilatation may be easily obtained the day of the operation. Elevation of intraocular pressure may be easily monitored if the rules of not opening a very soft lens too soon are respected. For optimum results, some rules must be followed. All patients that undergo an anterior capsulotomy must have both of their pupils fully dilated with phenylephrine 10% + cyclopentolate 1%. From the day of the capsulotomy, patients are kept on either topical or oral indomethacin and the IOP is monitored by checking the eye pressure every two hours. A 10-15-mm Hg pressure rise may be treated eventually with timoptic 0.50% drops and acetazolamide. We seldom need a manitol infusion at surgery to lower eye pressure and have always been able to perform surgery through a clear cornea.

Another advantage of the pulsed YAG capsulotomy is that one may shape it as desired, according to the lens to be inserted or according to whether or not the surgeon wants an "in the bag" lens implantation. If so, the anterior capsulotomy will be as large as possible or have a visible inferior flap with which to put the inferior loop in the bag. The capsulotomy must be rapidly done to avoid corneal drying and must be coaxial to avoid chances of iris damage.

Sometimes it may be difficult to exactly locate the anterior capsule. A very simple way is to trap plasma bubbles in the anterior cortex in two or three shots and to shoot on the bubble; the escape of the bubble in the anterior chamber is proof that the anterior capsule is really being opened.

The nucleus itself and cortical material may be amenable to softening by pulsed, Nd YAG laser bursts. A hard nucleus may be shot even inside the bag, the phacoemulsification may be facilitated, which represents a significant advance, making any lens available for this procedure. To be really efficient and to not use too many bursts to adequately fragment the nucleus, higher power densities are required and we usually soften the nucleus with the picosecond YAG laser, working the laser at a six-millijoule output energy level. With too low a power density, it would take too many bursts to adequately fragment the nucleus. One special application of nuclear softening would be prior to pars plana lensectomy and before vitrectomy, in the case of a hard lens that would present problems for phacoemulsification when the surgeon does not have the option of converting to a larger incision and expressing the nucleus.

Safety Considerations and Side Effects

Respecting the basic rules of laser delivery in 2,500 anterior capsulotomies, we observed no modification in the endothelial cell count immediately post-laser. IOP has always been well controlled. The rate of post-op CME was similar to that of the usual ECCE procedure (0.75%), and the rate of retinal detachment post-operatively was extremely low (0.2%). Phakoanaphylactic reactions have never been observed, but all patients underwent indomethacin treatment prior to and two weeks after surgery.

Discission of Secondary Membranes in Pseudophakic Patients

One of the most practical uses of the pulsed, Nd YAG laser at this time has been the discission of secondary membranes in pseudophakic patients (Figs. 17-25).

The ability to leave the capsule intact at surgery and to do a laser discission at any time after surgery, as needed, has significantly changed our management of the posterior capsule. Laser capsulotomy is a safe and effective procedure. Depending on the thickness of the membrane and the residual cortex, a range of from one or two to over 200 laser bursts are necessary to obtain almost instantaneous recovery of vision. In terms of safety to the intraocular lens, pseudophakic patients should definitively be operated on using the laser beam coaxially and dissociating the plane of operator focus from the YAG beam. The YAG burst must explode deeper than the posterior capsule, and only the anterior reflexion of the shock wave will be employed to open the posterior capsule. This is easily obtained by adjusting the eyepieces of the slit lamp to plus one diopter from the operator refraction.

For a posterior capsulotomy behind a PCL with the picosecond YAG laser, the output energy must be attenuated down to three to five millijoules; this is insured by the interposition of attenuating filters. More security is provided by using a +60 diopters Abraham lens. This concentrates the laser beam so much that the risk of hitting the lens is miniscule. From my experience in over 2,000 posterior capsulotomies in pseudophakic patients, 52 have been accidentally marked, most of them by training doctors who did not yet know how to handle the laser properly. There are definite differences between types of IOLs in terms of hardness of surface, material, and purity of materials and in how the lens itself might be affected by the laser. Besides, aspherical lenses, which do not seem to be as comfortable optically as the others, are far easier to leave untouched when performing a posterior capsulotomy.

From our experience, the pitting of an IOL has never been a clinical problem. The restitution of vision is immediate anyway, and in over five years follow-up, I noted no intolerance, reaction, or late deterioration of the lens related to laser marking of the PMMA.

With the pico-pulsed, modulated YAG laser, it is not necessary to diverge the beam as much as with a nanosecond one. Therefore, posterior capsulotomy may be performed even through small pupils. Furthermore, it is sometimes better to center the first hole on the posterior capsule prior to dilating the pupil and then do the complete capsulotomy.

Several techniques can reduce the potential of complications such as pitting of the IOL, inflammatory reactions, increased IOP, or CME. To reduce the potential of pitting the IOL, the coaxial position and a +45 to +60 diopter contact lens is by far the safest. It avoids the long, oblique, destructive funnel that may affect the lens.

Posterior capsulotomies in pseudophakic patients with anterior chamber or iris plane lenses do not need protective adjustment of the eyepieces of the slit lamp. In case of PCL, one should adjust the eyepieces in such a way that the burst will occur deeper in the vitreous. The breakdown will be easily seen by the "tell tale" blue spark. Then the beam is moved slightly forward. The second burst will occur just behind the capsule and the anterior diffusion of the shock wave will easily open the capsule. The more tense the capsule, the fewer the necessary bursts. In fact, I often find the laser posterior capsulotomy easier to achieve (one or two shots only) in posterior chamber lenses that keep the capsule smooth and tense.

One must also be aware of the axis of the capsulary tension and perform the laser capsulotomy perpendicular to the tension lines. This will considerably reduce the number of laser shots necessary to achieve a good opening.

Up to now, there have been no methods of avoiding CME. Delaying the posterior capsulotomy for as long as possible after surgery may reduce the incidence. We recommend not trapping vitreous in too narrow a capsulotomy. The capsule has to be holed or cross-opened, but not cut square, to avoid flaps falling inside the vitreous.

Avoidance of CME, Increase of IOP, and Inflammatory Reactions

In the case of a fine capsule when the capsulotomy can be achieved with a few bursts and in one session, no post-treatment is required, and the restitution of the vision is immediate. Under these conditions, we never observed any increase in the IOP or CME.

When much cortex remains in the center of the capsule, many bursts may be necessary to open it. It is useless and dangerous, in our opinion, to try and achieve the operation in one session. Complications such as inflammatory reactions, flare in AC, increased IOP, and, in some cases, transient CME may occur. We find it much safer to process in several (two to five) sessions, keeping the patient's eye under treatment with mydriatics, timoptic, and anti-inflammatory drops (indomethacin and/or prednisone). According to how rapidly the lens material is reabsorbed, the next session will be scheduled.

For example, Figs. 22A-C show especially heavy lens material. Five sessions, with 100 to 200 bursts each, were necessary to clear up the pupillary area. One week separated the first from the second session, and three to four days passed between the remaining three sessions. In respecting these precautions, we minimized the possible complications (increased IOP and inflammatory reactions, etc.). Anyway, in these cases, it is normal to observe a temporarily increased IOP for 24 to 48 hours, usually not exceeding 10mm Hg.

Cutting Small Adhesions Directly Attached or Near IOLs

It is readily possible to cut small adhesions directly attached to and/or near intraocular lenses. Cleaning out an inflammatory membrane coating the anterior face of the lens is easily achieved without marking the lens. Both the posterior plasma shield and the hard structure of the lens protect against diffusion of the shock wave. The thickened cornea, due to endothelial malfunction, is likely to absorb a lot of energy from the laser beam prior to the focal point, substantially weakening the burst. Besides, the precise focusing of the aiming beam is very difficult to achieve in these cases.

When an iridolens synechiae is ruptured, resulting in a slight, pigmented or blood flare in the anterior chamber, it is safer and more efficient to wait for the flare to spontaneously clear up and lase again on clear media a few hours later.

Posterior Capsulotomies in Aphakic Patients Without an IOL

Posterior capsulotomies in aphakic patients without an IOL are certainly the easiest operations available with the pulsed YAG lasers, whatever the site and the thickness of the remaining lens material and whatever the cause of the secondary cataract. If residual lens material is present, the same precautions and treatment are recommended (Figs. 26-30).

Safety Considerations and Side Effects

In over 3,500 posterior capsulotomies (pseudophakos and aphakic), we have not observed significant or unexpected complications. Three percent of the lenses have been marked, but, as said before, without influence on improvement of visual acuity or on transparency of the IOL. In five years follow-up, no intolerance to a pitted IOL was noticed.

Serial endothelial cell counting has not demonstrated any early or late change.

Intraocular pressure rise, when it occurred, was always transient and was not higher than 15 mmHg above baseline and was fully controlled in all cases with medical therapy. Since following the rules of "not spreading too much lens material at once" and keeping the patient under observation and on anti-inflammatory treatment, we have observed less tendency toward an increased IOP than in past years.

A light flare in the anterior chamber is constantly observed as soon as some cortex is spread and floats into the anterior chamber. Local corticosteroid, mydriatic, and indomethacin have been effective in preventing any long-lasting (more than three days) or heavy inflammatory reactions.

The real incidence of CME caused by laser treatment appears to be low, although Robert Sinskey reported one case of transient CME following a posterior capsulotomy. Routine fluorescein angiography done after laser treatment is not always possible before laser treatment due to an opaque capsule. We did not notice the onset of CME post-laser in any patients with previously performed, normal angiography. Most often, the immediate and permanent restitution of the vision is a second proof of this fact.

The incidence of retinal detachment following pico laser posterior capsulotomy is less than one out of 3,000, and the relation has only been proven in that one case.

Iridocapsular and Iridopseudophakos Adhesions

Iridocapsular and iridopseudophakos adhesions are readily performed with the YAG laser. Slight bleeding may be expected each time a vascularized synechiae is lased, but it always cleared up in a few hours. Mydriatrics and anti-inflammatory treatment must be given to reduce chances of recurrences. But, in more than 800 cases of cutting synechiae, the rate of recurrence is still about 22%. However, if inflammatory adhesions recur, re-treatment with the laser is always possible (Figs. 31-33).

Pupillary block glaucoma and rupture of inflammatory membranes in aphakic patients are among the very practical uses of the pulsed, Nd YAG laser. From our experience, the majority of these patients will present with a red eye, flat anterior chamber, and hazy cornea. It is mandatory to clear up the cornea and try to obtain at least some distance between the posterior cornea and the block. For this purpose, a very rapid 25% manitol infusion (500 Ml infused within 15 minutes) will produce a transient dehydration of the vitreous and permit the formation of an anterior chamber and some clearing of the cornea. Topical glycerine may also help (Figs. 34-36). In cases where the cornea has been cleared up, the effect is spectacular and immediate. As soon as a hole has been formed in the iris or the inflammatory membrane, the anterior chamber will deepen and the intraocular pressure, already lowered by medical treatment, will remain normal if two conditions are respected:

1—In cases of mechanical, aphakic, pupillary block with multiple, separate posterior chambers vitreous pouches, each of them must be laser-opened; otherwise, there is a high incidence of recurrence.

2—In case of pupillary block due to inflammatory membrane, there is a high incidence of recurrence, even with anti-inflammatory treatment.

Safety considerations and side effects. In nearly 300 patients treated for these conditions, the incidence of corneal pitting is very high (40%) due to the flat anterior chamber. Post-laser modifications in endothelial cell counting cannot be studied since it is impossible to perform pre-laser and post-laser counts on these swollen corneas. Bleeding of the iris occurred each time a burst exploded in the iris, but the bleeding has always disappeared in less than two hours. No retinal detachment can be related to this treatment, even in the cases where deep aqueous humor pouches were trapped in the vitreous.

Pupillary Ascensions

Updrawn pupils may be opened in aphakic patients. The more tense the iris, the fewer the necessary bursts. Often, better tension on the pupil is obtained by attempting maximal dilatation with phenylephrine 10% and cyclopentolate (Fig. 37). The beam may be used coaxially or laterally since, as long as no IOL is present, there is no danger. The argon laser can be of help in opening the pupil by directly cutting the iris or by using non-perforating, low energy. Longer-duration argon burns will tense the iris for YAG treatment. However, if the picosecond YAG shock wave is more powerful in terms of power density, it is far more limited in thickness and expansion of the shock than the nano and, therefore, as far as an iris is concerned, its pigmented layers will absorb most of the light passing through if optical breakdown does not occur. This is why I prefer the free-running, nanosecond, pulsed YAG or the argon laser to the pico YAG for any iridotomy.

Safety Considerations and Side Effects. The only complications that have been observed in treating pupillary ascension were transient bleeding of the iris and the failure to achieve iridotomy when the iris was not tense enough.

Attempts have been made to pop out iris cysts or epithelial downgrowths. For this operation, in the few cases we did, immediate success was obtained, whatever the position of the beam. However, when dealing with epithelial downgrowth, laser treatment cannot remove the cause and does not cancel the indications for surgery.

Releasing iris adhesions to a normal lens or posterior iris synechiae in uveitis on phakic patients must not be attempted unless the surgeon is perfectly capable of locating the anterior capsule of the lens to avoid opening it. However, the risk of damaging the lens (even if adjusting the laser beam anteriorly and shooting only in the coaxial position) is too high to consider it as one of the reasonable, pulsed YAG laser indications.

Howard C. Cohn, M.D.
William Whalen, M.D.

THE PICOSECOND YAG LASER IN GLAUCOMA TREATMENT

6

The YAG laser may be used quite successfully, either alone or as an adjunct to the argon laser, in the treatment of certain glaucoma conditions. These include pupillary block glaucoma, peripheral anterior synechiae, occluded glaucoma fistulas, congenital glaucoma, and creation of a graded trabeculectomy procedure.

Iridotomies may be made with the pulsed, picosecond YAG laser irrespective of iris color. However, because of its nonthermal effect, iris bleeding tends to occur more often than with the argon laser. Sometimes a transient hyphema is produced. It is rare for significant bleeding to occur, but the major problem is simply practical: if enough microscopic blood is suspended in the aqueous humor, effective delivery of the YAG beam may become impossible and the patient will have to return for retreatment. An additional problem is that, when shooting at the iris periphery in an eye with a narrow iridocorneal angle, the corneal endothelium tends to whiten with each laser shot due to the anterior reflection of the shock wave, even if perfectly focused on the iris. This whitening is temporary, but can hinder the view for further laser delivery.

Our procedure of choice in phakic eyes is still the argon laser iridotomy with an Abraham-type converging contact lens, even for the light blue-grey iris that may be the most difficult to perforate. Actually, it is not perforation that most often poses a problem, but enlarging the iridotomy to an adequate, functional size. The iris stroma seems to absorb the laser energy, but no vaporization of tissue is produced. (The futility of trying to put a hole in a sponge with a water gun comes to mind.) We routinely leave these cases for four to six weeks, at which time secondary enlargement by argon laser is easier due to pigment proliferation. Yet, on occasion, adequate enlargement is still not possible, and it is these cases where the YAG laser may be used on the area pre-treated by argon laser. We use the Abraham iridotomy lens with the mode-locked, YAG, picosecond laser without problems, although special lenses for the YAG laser are available.

Isolated spot peripheral, anterior goniosynechiae may be liberated with the YAG laser. The goal is not to recover function of the trabecular meshwork to which the iris adhered, but to help prevent further, circumferential sticking of the iris to the angle structures.

An especially exciting application of the pulsed YAG laser is in re-opening occluded glaucoma fistulas.[1] This can sometimes be achieved with the argon laser, but pigmented tissue is required,[2] whereas the YAG laser works equally well on all tissues, pigmented or not. And, in our experience, occlusion of trabeculectomies most often occurs by formation of an opaque non-pigmented membrane that either completely occludes the opening or seals the underside of the scleral flap to the surrounding sclera. YAG picolaser shots can often cut through this membrane and free the scleral flap, reestablishing subconjunctival filtration if significant conjunctival scarring has not also occurred.

Another use of the YAG laser is the creation of a graded trabeculectomy procedure. A thin scleral flap can be fashioned at surgery and then sutured more tightly than usual, helping to reform the anterior chamber in the immediate post-operative period. Then, part of the flap can be shot open progressively to give the desired degree of filtration.

Other practical applications of the YAG laser in glaucoma include laser goniotomy for congenital glaucoma (pediatrics chapter).

The following uses are still experimental, but will be discussed here because of their interesting potential.

The YAG laser has two possible applications in open-angle glaucoma: In open-angle glaucoma, argon laser trabeculoplasty has been shown to be effective in lowering intraocular pressure [3] by increasing outflow facility.[4] Trabeculoplasty is felt to produce its effect by opening trabecular spaces between two burns, by concentric constriction of the trabecular ring, by opening Schlemm's canal, or by tensing the meshwork as in the action of pilocarpine.

Thermal YAG burns may be placed on the trabecular meshwork in exactly the same manner that argon laser treatment would be given. However, characteristics of the burns produced would not necessarily be similar. The 488 to 545-nanometer wavelength of the argon laser is preferentially absorbed by hemoglobin, generating thermal effects at the point of energy absorption. However, hemoglobin and pigmented tissues at nearby wavelengths are relatively more transparent for the 1064-nanometer YAG light. Therefore, YAG laser energy passes deeper into such tissues since less is absorbed and fewer thermal effects can be expected for similar power levels and spots sizes. Even increasing the power of a cw YAG laser would not insure duplication of the argon laser trabecular burn, which has been shown to be so clinically effective. Whether or not thermal YAG trabecular burns may have any advantages over argon laser treatment cannot be answered at the present time.

Pulsed YAG shots offer a completely different approach. The nonthermal mini-explosion of the optical breakdown may be delivered to the anterior chamber angle with the aim of mechanically disrupting the trabecular meshwork. Two levels of treatment are theoretically possible:

1. A through-and-through hole may be opened from the anterior chamber into the subconjunctival space, establishing a glaucoma fistula on a completely closed eye. We have attempted this exciting possibility with the mode-locked, picosecond YAG laser on four patients before trabeculectomy, but without success. Several hundred shots were aimed at a point on the anterior trabecular meshwork just behind Schwalbe's line.

2. A second possibility is producing varying degrees of internal trabeculotomy either by just disrupting superficial meshwork or by actually making holes through to Schlemm's canal.

However, results of early studies to date have been inconclusive. We have no evidence yet that any benefit is obtained by this type of trabecular treatment.

Safety Considerations

The most serious complication of doing an iridotomy with the "cold" YAG laser can occur in phakic eyes if the lens capsule is inadvertently opened. This could produce a lens induced phacoanaphylactic uveitis and accelerater cataract formation. For this reason, we do not recommend doing YAG laser iridotomies in phakic eyes, with the exception of the occasional, absolute failure of the argon laser method. However, (as discussed in chapter five), in aphakic eyes with pupillary block or an occluded pupil, for example, the YAG laser may be easily used.

Reference

1. Cohn, H, Aron-Rosa, D: YAG laser reopening of blocked trabeculectomy (in press). Amer. J. Ophthal.
2. Van Buskirk, E: Reopening filtration fistulas with the argon laser; Amer. J. Ophthal. 94, I, 1982.
3. Wise, J: Long term control of adult open angle glaucoma by argon laser treatment; Ophthalmology 88:197–202, 1981.
4. Wilensky, J, Jampol, L: Laser therapy for open angle glaucoma. Ophthalmology 88:213–217, 1981.

Danièle S. Aron-Rosa, M.D.
Elisabeth Jeanneau, M.D.

THE PICOSECOND YAG LASER IN VITREOUS SURGERY

7

One of the most useful applications of YAG laser surgery is its use on posterior vitreous membrane and strands or traction bands. One may readily cut bands coming through or behind the pupil. The operation is safe and easy to perform when the traction is tense. In many cases of CME, with vitreous traction bands coming up from the posterior pole to the corneal wound or to the pupillary borders, both cutting them with the YAG laser and subjecting the patient to anti-inflammatory treatment often resulted in improvement of vision and resolution of the CME. Patients were controlled by pre- and post-laser fluorescein angiography. However, the improvement of visual acuity is not as immediate as in posterior capsulotomy, and a minimum two to three-week delay is to be expected before reaching a definite result. Most of these membranes were easily cut anteriorly without a contact lens. Eventually, to shoot in the vitreous, an Abraham-type iridotomy lens may be used (Figs. 38-43).

Retinovitreal traction bands and preretinal membranes require a triple-mirror, fundus-type lens and topical anesthetic to precisely locate the traction. Because we avoid draining subretinal fluid at retinal detachment surgery, we often release the traction bands holding an RD, making it mobile and, thus, facilitating the no-drain procedure. Also, one of the most useful applications of the pulsed YAG laser is to release a single traction band, which keeps a horseshoe tear open. One can also cut off the flap of the tear before retinal surgery when a retinal detachment is present, or after argon laser photocoagulation around the hole when the retina is flat. In case of a very limited retinal detachment, the section of the traction of the flap makes the Lincoff balloon procedure easier and more efficient. According to the nature of the traction, from four to several hundred laser bursts may be required.

In dealing with traction bands, the most difficult step for the surgeon is to find the right orientation for laser delivery. The most efficient way is to cut perpendicular to the direction of maximum traction. However, this is not always possible when the safety of the retina and lens are considered. Also it is possible to work on *encapsulated foreign bodies,* peeling membranes off by laser before surgical extraction. Breaking up *floaters* may be a possibility, although mobile formations will be moved around more than exploded by the shock wave.

Safety Considerations and Side Effects

One must work with the laser beam in the coaxial position as much as possible, which is the usual position, in any case, for a good fundus view (normal position for argon laser treatments). The security distance for the retina is far less than one millimeter with the pico YAG. As long as optical breakdown is reached in air, it will always occur in aqueous or vitreous. And, in the case of seven to eight-train, 30-picosecond pulses, a very rapid plasma screen is generated so that 88 to 90% of the incident laser beam is absorbed or scattered in the breakdown process (in vitro measurements). Although the level of irradiation on the retina posterior to the optical breakdown point is reduced, 8 to 12% still reaches the posterior pole.

But, in dealing with energy and power densities, at the thresholds required for optical breakdown, the mechanisms of damage are related to the absorption characteristics of the tissue and the power density of the laser pulse where it impinges on the tissue. Considering these facts and experimental studies on the generation and diffusion in the vitreous of both acoustical (elastic) and shock (inelastic) waves, we consider one millimeter from the retina to be a safe distance. However, improvement in new laser devices may allow the exact safe distance to be computerized and calculated, given the difficulty and inaccuracy of the ophthalmologist working in the vitreous with his eyes alone and not his hands.

The tissue anterior to (upstream from) the focal point will not be protected by the plasma screen and is fully exposed to the free diffusion of both acoustical and shock pressure waves. Therefore, one must remain at least one millimeter behind the lens to be safe, as demonstrated by pathologic studies. Using the laser beam from the lateral position when dealing with the anterior vitreous can increase the chances of damaging the lens. The coaxial position will definitely offer more security.

Side effects that may be observed are related to the patient's pathology. Local hemorrhages were seen after the section of vitreous membranes containing blood vessels. More importantly, intravitreal hemorrhage may occur when a larger blood vessel is cut off. Argon laser or YAG thermal coagulation before shock-wave cutting of a vascularized membrane is theoretically possible, but, in practice, we have found that prior coagulation is no assurance that bleeding will not occur anyway.

In general, we do not consider diabetic, proliferative retinopathy one of the best indications for the presently available devices.

Inflammatory membranes recurred after treatment in 20% of cases and had to be retreated four times, on the average, but isolated, tense traction bands do not reform in our experience of 300 cases. Preretinal membranes may sometimes be released when stretched from point to point on the retina, but when they are stuck to the retina, they cannot be treated by available YAG lasers because of the danger of retinal injury. No CME or change in the endothelial cell count or permanent modifications in the IOP was observed in treated patients. Each time (5/300) a local hemorrhage did occur, it reabsorbed within five days. We noted no retinal detachment or retinal hole caused by the laser.

Having had the opportunity of spending several years following up a physicist who received an accidental YAG picopulsed laser shot on his macula, we noted no necrosis, swelling, or RD, and vision remained unchanged at 20/60. Fluorescein angiography has shown a limited fenestration of the pigment epithelium without CME.

From Experimental Retinal Shots (See Pathology)

Pathologic studies performed one to 15 days after a single laser shot showed: at 3.5 millijoules output in a burst of seven pulses, clear, limited tissue destruction without perforation of the retina and without hemorrhages. The internal limiting membrane was not ruptured, and swelling of the surrounding four layers of cells present on the eye were removed one day after laser treatment. No necrosis of the surrounding tissue and no swelling of the normal, surrounding cells were seen on the eye, which was removed on the seventh day. When the output energy reached 6.5 millijoules, the retina was perforated and hemorrhages had spread into the vitreous. On the eye, removed one day after laser application to the retina, the internal limiting membrane was ruptured and heavy, but limited, exudation was present under the retina. The choroid and sclera were normal.

On the second eye, removed 15 days after laser application, the perforation of the entire thickness of the retina was comparable to the previous patient. No adhesive scar was visible, the retina was flat, and exudation had disappeared. The surrounding cells around the retinal perforation appeared normal. Fluorescein angiography before enucleation showed dry lesions without evidence of CME.

Pulsed YAG lasers may permit safe, precise surgery, even in phakic patients, if safety distances, both to the lens and the retina, are respected. In case of vascularized traction bands and diabetic retinopathy, pulsed YAG laser treatment must be considered risky and employed with great caution, if at all.

Jean-Jacques Aron, M.D.

THE PICOSECOND YAG LASER IN PEDIATRIC OPHTHALMOLOGY

8

Potential applications of Nd pulsed YAG lasers in pediatric ophthalmology are similar to those of adults and are, in some ways, more extensive. Due to the frequent necessity of performing the laser session under general anesthesia, it is more comfortable, for certain indications, to mount a laser on a microscope or to a slit lamp, allowing one to treat a prone patient. A production model of a microscope laser is not yet available.

Over 500 children up to 12 years of age have already undergone YAG laser treatment with the usual prototype. In infants and young children (younger than four years of age), the sessions have been performed under Ketamine by intramuscular injection with the anesthesiologist always present. The injection may be repeated without danger as soon as the eyes start to swing up. Both anterior and posterior capsulotomies were easily performed either in traumatic or congenital cataract. "Softening" of a hard nucleus has proven to be very useful just prior to pars plana or anterior lensectomy.

One of the most practical uses of the pulsed Nd YAG laser at this time has been treatment of heavy lens material remaining after either *congenital* or *traumatic cataract surgery*. Considering the great ability of the child's eye to reabsorb lens material, fewer sessions are required than in adult patients. However, full dilatation of the pupil, topical steroids, and indomethacin drops treatment have always been associated with the laser sessions.

Total laser treatment of a *cataract* by opening the anterior capsule and letting the lens material resorb must not be considered the best approach to removal of a congenital cataract unless a permanent contraindication to general anesthesia is present. The results and complications are comparable to those of the "old time" needling of the lens. The only advantages are that the technique is noninvasive and it is possible to progressively open the anterior capsule over several weeks to prevent the complications caused by the swelling of an already soft cortex and nucleus (Figs. 44-46).

Congenital glaucoma, with a cleared cornea and a Barkan-type membrane, may be efficiently treated by laser without complications and with very positive results. No recurrence or readherence of the Barkan's membrane tends to occur.

Although a newborn child is not perfectly comfortable at the slit lamp and will require possible modifications of the device, laser goniotomy has proven to be a perfectly safe and efficient technique.

Follow-up of these few patients did not exceed two years. Its advantages are the possibility of repeating the treatment as many times as required and the fact that the entire 360° angle is accessible, which is not the case with a single goniotomy incision.

Both *vitreous traction bands* and avascular, congenital, vitreous formations have readily been successfully treated with the YAG laser.

Initial experimental work has shown that the pulsed Nd YAG laser is a relatively safe instrument that provides a new approach to many common and rare ophthalmic diseases in children. As soon as the microscope-mounted laser is available for more easily treating infants and children under general anesthesia, the indications for treatment will expand.

R. Birngruber, M.D., Ph.D.
B. P. Gabel, M.D.
K. P. Boergen, M.D.
H. R. Zink, M.D.

THE GERMAN EXPERIENCE IN YAG LASER SURGERY SIDE EFFECTS USING ULTRASHORT, PULSED, NEODYNIUM YAG LASERS IN INTRAOCULAR MICROSURGERY

9

Side effects of two different laser systems producing nanosecond and picosecond pulses were compared. The Q-switched, nanosecond laser system (LASAG) was tested in two modifications. The mode-locked, monomode, picosecond laser (MEDITEC) had provided a constant output energy of six millijoules in bursts of seven pulses of 25 picoseconds each.

Working in reproducible parameters in different eye segments of chinchilla grey rabbits, side effects on the cornea, iris, lens, and retina were studied.

1. Iridectomies on a normal iris are not possible with the picosecond YAG laser. No corneal damage or cataract was seen.

   Iridotomies are nicely produced with the nano Q-switched laser by using a special contact lens, and a five-millijoule output energy allowed to perforate the iris. Thermal coagulation of the iris was necessary to avoid bleeding by using the ten-millisecond pulses produced by the microruptor. Without using the contact lens, corneal damage was constantly seen.

   Acute iridectomies (Fig. 47A) showed a large defect of pigment epithelium around the hole, and the lens anterior capsule behind was locally and irreversibly opacified.

   The eye, removed four weeks after the nanosecond laser application, showed wide enlargement of the iridectomy with stromal atrophy and pigment dispersion in the anterior chamber (Figs. 47B, 47C), which never occurs in human nano YAG laser iridectomies.

2. *Anterior capsulotomies* with the *picosecond, monomode, mode-locked YAG laser* do not necessitate use of a contact lens. The splitting of the anterior capsule is successful at a rate of 100%. In focusing or defocusing the aiming beam, one may vary the size of the destruction by 90 microns or more on the surface and from 0.2 mm to 0.5 mm in depth. In doing capsulotomies, we noted no damage to the cornea, even when the beam was not focused in the coaxial position (Figs. 48A-C, 49A, B).

   Using the Q-switched laser without a contact lens, capsulotomies induced cell necrosis of the corneal *epithelium* in many cases. The side effects were reversible in a few days and were totally avoided by using the contact lens.

   After nano- or picosecond-induced posterior or anterior capsulotomies, no damage on the retina was seen either by clinical examination or at fluorescein angiography.

3. In splitting vitreous strands, we tried to appreciate the security distance to be respected to avoid retinal side effects. Distances between vitreous focal spots and the retina were measured through a micrometer screw-system fixed at the top of the slit lamp (Fig. 50).

   Using the Q-switched nanosecond laser, side effects depended on both output energy and focus-to-retina distance. Lesions of three millimeters appeared when the output energy was at 1.5 millijoules (which is under the optical breakdown level). When reaching the output energy for optical breakdown (2.5 to 3.5 millijoules, according to whether the laser works multimode or near to monomode), the retina could be approached to within one millimeter more without being damaged. Power levels below the optical breakdown threshold produced subretinal bleedings and rupture of the retina. Using the monomode modification of the nanosecond YAG clearly appeared as a possibility to reduce side effects on the retina.

   Mode-locked, monomode, picosecond lasers may produce retinal damage at a distance of between one and 1.5 mm. The optical breakdown was reached in all cases. In contrast to Q-switched lasers, there is no graduation in retinal damage, and as long as the output energy was not graduated, the lesion is a local retinal rupture with hemorrhage (Figs. 51A-C).

In summary (Fig. 52):

- Iridectomies are not possible in rabbits using the picosecond laser;
- Nanosecond-induced iridectomies show large involvement of the pigment epithelium around the hole, together with an enlargement of the primary laser-induced effect and a local, irreversible opacification of the anterior lens capsule;
- Neither anterior nor posterior capsulotomy induced retinal lesions;
- Corneal lesions were never seen with the picosecond YAG laser when working in the anterior chamber. In rabbits, they were constant with the nanosecond laser but could be easily avoided by using a contact lens;
- In working in the vitreous, the security distance to be respected to avoid retinal side effects is slightly shorter with the picosecond YAG laser than with the nanosecond, and the induced lesion is narrower and more limited in the picosecond laser-induced lesion; and
- Working under the optical breakdown threshold is far more dangerous than working at the threshold levels, which stresses the importance of the plasma shield formation. It is less dangerous to dial an output energy of from three to four millijoules with the nanosecond than to work at one to two millijoules.

Richard D. Keates, M.D.

Q-SWITCHED NANOSECOND PULSED ND YAG LASERS

10

There are approximately 40,000 YAG laser rods in the United States today. Of this large number, probably less than 25 are being used at the time of this writing for short pulse ophthalmic delivery systems. These few YAG lasers have been available in the United States for investigational purposes for less than one year. Although ophthalmologists are quite familiar with argon lasers, and somewhat familiar with CO_2 lasers, there has been very little experience with the unique low-energy pulses delivered by the various YAG configurations when membrane perforations are desired. It is also not uncommon in emerging technology to have significant differences of opinion. The early work of Aron-Rosa led her to construct and utilize a picosecond mode-locked Nd YAG system, while that of Fankhauser caused him to develop and utilize a Q-switched delivery system for the same purposes. In this book Aron-Rosa details the advantages of mode-locking. In this chapter I will attempt to explain my preference and techniques of Q-switch delivering of the energy.

Laser damage mechanisms include thermal, photochemical and mechanical mechanisms. The damage levels are achieved as a result of the combinations of pulse energy, time and focal area of the beam resulting in a specific power density. The unique characteristic of Nd YAG irradiation which makes it attractive for ophthalmology today is that of the mechanical effect caused by pressure waves if the proper configuration of the laser is attained. Although thermal effects may also be obtained with a YAG configuration and may be desirable, still little is known of the comparative effects of the YAG thermal effect as compared to the readily available argon thermal effects. In ophthalmology up to this time, there has not been the ability to cut selectively or rupture the non-pigmented membranes within the eye. The uniqueness of the Nd YAG laser is that, by the achievement of a threshold optical power density which causes electrostriction and diaelectric breakdown, it is easy to show optical breakdown. Optical breakdown appears as a small spark in gases and liquids by focusing the beam to a small enough spot. The breakdown, which is the ionization of the medium through intense electrical fields, results in the deposition of energy in the beam in the region of the breakdown. This generates acoustic waves that can probably account for the rupture of the target membranes. With the nano laser, I work above the optical breakdown level. Designing a system to cause optical breakdown and ruptured membranes in the eye—such as posterior capsules, specific configurations, or methods of delivery—must be considered. The two main methods being utilized today, as stated earlier, are the Q-switched nanosecond pulse and the picosecond mode-locked pulse. Both in their specific configurations can probably cause these membranes to be ruptured. The difference between the Q-switch and mode-lock is in the method of pulsing the laser. The Q-switch units use an electronic shutter commonly called a Pockels cell. The mode-lock units currently available use a passive dye cell.

Initially, I was unsure of which method was preferable; therefore, a prototype Nd YAG laser was constructed for use at The Ohio State University by American Medical Optics of Irvine California. This laser had both the ability to be Q-switched and mode-locked. It was initially designed to emulate that of the Q-switched laser as utilized by Fankhauser and the mode-locked laser as utilized by Aron-Rosa in terms of the same time, envelope, and spot size. It contained a specific Nd YAG laser and helium neon guide laser beam, expanding optics, a slit lamp for delivery of the beam, a mechanism for delivering the beam from the lasers to the moving slit lamp electronics including laser power supplies, laser energy monitoring devices, safety interlocks and a suitable housing.

Initial clinical results utilizing this prototype laser in posterior capsulotomies revealed that, while both were clinically effective, there were cases where patients who had started with mode-locking who required Q-switching to open effectively the membrane as higher power densities were needed than were available with the mode-locked system. In addition, the dye in the cells ages and ultimately becomes ineffective and must be replaced, which is not necessary with the Q-switched system. It is also less expensive to construct a Q-switched laser, and probably less expensive to maintain. There did not appear clinically to be any difference in the safety factors or safety ranges in my initial series between the two lasers. Based on the above was my feeling that the Q-switched method with nanosecond pulsing provided an effective clinical instrument; a second production model Q-switched Nd YAG laser was constructed.

Characteristics of Clinical Model Nd YAG Laser

The clinical model constructed consisted of the following characteristics: A wave length of 1064 nm energy dose of from 1 to 20 millijoules, pulse duration of 20 nanoseconds, spot size of 50 microns. The resultant configuration is shown (Figs. 53, 54). Upon powering up, all interlocks are activated and the shutters closed. The Nd YAG laser may be fired with the shutter closed to verify power settings; a helium neon laser shutter is opened to allow visualization for aiming of the YAG beam as the two beams travel in a coaxial path. Power delivered to the patient can be adjusted using attenuators. Since all of these devices at the present time are investigational all clinical use must be under established protocols approved by the Bureau of Radiological Health and also by human research or institutional research boards.

Clinical Experience

There are many potential clinical applications of the Nd YAG laser but most of the clinical experience is with relatively few conditions. The following will detail my clinical experience and philosophy toward the use of this modality. Perusal of the clinical experience of others is provided in the Bibliography at the end of the book.

Posterior Capsulotomies

The most common application has been in the use of posterior capsulotomies in the aphakic or pseudophakic patients. Increasing use of extracapsular cataract extraction along with an increasing tendency to leave the posterior capsules initially intact at the end of surgery has resulted in an increased number of opaque posterior capsules at a later date. Although these numbers will vary depending upon the surgeon and the technique utilized, it would probably be safe to estimate these are at least 30% over a long period of time. The noninvasive characteristics of the YAG laser provide an excellent modality for treating or opening these membranes.

The commonly seen form of posterior capsule in the United States today is a thin membrane with secondary pearls or epithelial cells across the visual axis. Prior to treating these with the YAG laser one should determine the visual axis prior to dilation as it is possible to be off center with the laser as well as with a knife and scalpel. If contact lenses have been worn by the patient it is best to try and leave the contact lens off to reduce the chance of corneal edema which may interfere with the laser beam. A 3- to 5-mm central opening is desired. The typical membrane may be readily opened by utilizing one to two millijoule pulses. After dilatation the patient is positioned at the slit lamp delivery system. The helium neon beam, which is coincident with the YAG beam, is focused on the membrane. The patient requires no other medication or anesthetic. A central shot is fired. If this power level is effective a series of shots are delivered working up and down and left and right in a cross pattern across the last cut edge, gradually expanding the opening to the desired size. If the initial settings is not effective, one can turn up the power to two millijoules; if there are dense fibrotic bands higher power levels may be necessary. I have rarely had to go over three millijoules for most aphakic membranes. You should not try to cut flaps of capsule as these may swing back and forth in the surgeon's way and require many more shots to open the capsule effectively. In most aphakic membranes I have not found the need for the use of a contact lens either to steady the eye or help concentrate or focus the beam. The tighter or the more taut the capsule, the easier it is to open. The number of shots required will depend on the energy level; at low energy levels, fewer than 50 shots are usually required. Although fewer shots may be needed with higher energy/higher millijoule settings, it is a general feeling to use the lowest power setting to do the job as a safety precaution (Figs. 55-60).

In those cases, with the addition of an intraocular lens, the need for a detailed technique becomes more important to avoid possible damage to the intraocular lens. The closer the opaque membrane is to the intraocular lens, the more crucial the technique becomes. Such methods as offsetting the relationship between the helium neon beam and the YAG beam may be utilized to increase the safety. In this method, for example, one diopter may be added to the oculars over the clinician's prescription so as to cause the apparent focus of the red beam to be closer to the physician. The YAG beam, however, stays in the same position so that when the physician thinks he is focusing on the membrane with the red beam the YAG beam is one diopter behind. This slight bit of offset (.3 mm) allows for effective opening of the membrane and less chance of danger or pitting the intraocular lens. It is highly recommended that a one millijoule or less setting be utilized with intraocular lenses, particularly in those cases of posterior chamber lenses. It is also important not to fire repeatedly in the exact same position as this may increase the chance of damage to the IOL. There are definite differences between the types of IOLs in the ease with which marking may occur. The harder the IOL (the higher molecular weight) the harder it is to mark, particularly at low millijoule levels. Any time the millijoule level is increased—most noticeably at the 5 level with focusing at the level of the surface of the IOL—a mark on the lens may be caused. Marks or pits vary greatly from lens to lens in that they may be just small surface pits or in some cases almost disc-like in appearance. This may depend on stress marks on the IOL itself as to the definite characteristics of the mark. Although I have not seen visual effects or decrease in visual acuity caused by such marks, there certainly is the potential danger of this occurring and it should be kept uppermost at all times in the surgeon's mind (Figs. 61-64).

In most patients the procedure is accomplished quickly and comfortably with very little reaction noted. In those cases with a great number of pearls or some retained cortical material there may be more inflammation apparent. In these cases low dosage topical steroids may be indicated for the first week. In many patients no therapy appears to be indicated.

In regard to intraocular pressure some patients will show a temporary elevation following use of the laser. Whether this is caused by the shock bursts on the membrane causing inflammation or by liberated cellular material is still not quite clear. In one of our series, the average preoperative tension averaged 15, just after the procedure 17, at one week 16, and at one month 15 again. If the pressure should go up significantly, topical steroids and antiglaucoma medication, such as timoptic, may be indicated for a short time.

Complications of Posterior Capsulotomies

The opening of posterior capsules by invasive surgical means has been noted in the past to allow perhaps for certain complications of cataract surgery to occur such as the possibility of increased incidence of cystoid macular edema or conceivably retinal detachment. The use of the noninvasive laser capsulotomy may not cause such complications but it may not prevent their occurrence if they are specifically related to the opening of the capsule by any method. In my series of over 200 capsulotomies, one patient who had a small 1 mm capsulotomy performed and who had a history of high myopia and retinal detachment in the other eye developed an aphakic retinal detachment one month after laser discission (laser power density = 16 mj; working above optical breakdown level). A second patient developed lightning flashes and spots and floaters with a small hole approximately two and one-half months post laser discission. The second patient incidentally had had angiography after laser discission with a perfectly normal reading and normal appearance. Only one patient so far has developed known cystoid macular edema on followups either by me or the referring physicians. It is still too early in my series to evaluate the final effects on CME and retinal detachment. One may also cause small iris bleeders when opening dense membranes, particularly those in inflammatory cases where the membrane is close to the iris and it may be simply a shaking or vibration which breaks an adhesion and causes a small bleeder. A direct hit on the iris may also cause a small bleeder. Both of these are inconsequential and the bleeding stops immediately.

Preoperative Anterior Capsulotomies

Another potential indication is the use of the YAG to open the anterior capsule of the cataract in a circular or square fashion the day prior to planned extracapsular cataract extraction, which allows the surgeon to perform his capsulotomy the day before and to achieve an adequate and safe capsulotomy. In addition it may allow for hydration of the cortical material and theoretically allow for an easier mechanical washout the next day. It perhaps may allow for a softer nucleus if emulsification is being considered (Figs. 65-67).

In my opinion, current surgical technique in the United States including the use of substances such as sodium hyaluronate allow for a well defined and easily performed anterior capsulotomy at the time of surgery. This therefore obviates the need to perform the capsulotomy the day before and increase the chance of intraocular inflammation due to the procedure itself and the cortical stirring that occurs. In addition, it has not been proven to my satisfaction that nuclear softening is realistic at this time in terms of the power densities being utilized; however, if it can be proven that a nucleus can be softened in the bag so it is more amenable to emulsification, I am sure the technique would become widely used.

Anterior Chamber Adhesions

In a variety of clinical situations one may see either iris, capsule, or vitreous strands and adhesions which go to the wound and distort the pupil, or cause traction on intraocular lenses. These strands may also be implicated in the causation or prolongation of cystoid macular edema. The morbidity of invasive surgical management of these conditions is not inconsequential and therefore in some cases may delay intervention. The use of the noninvasive YAG pulses in these conditions should prove to be one of the prime considerations. Although these structures may be lysed by direct focusing, one should be careful not to strike the iris causing pain and possibly bleeding. It is usually best to try to lyse or cut these, or rupture these, by either going along the pupillary edge or up in the angle away from the iris if possible. To cut these effectively in the angle, one must use some form of gonio lens; it becomes important to use a lens which affords minimal distortion. I have used a Goldman type lens for this procedure. One can readily see the change in the focusing beam afforded by the peripheral astigmatism and perhaps by the lens itself. A series of lenses for this purpose has been developed by Prof. Fankhauser and also by Ocularus in Seattle, Washington. The lysis of these strands or bands is readily accomplished in either position utilizing somewhat higher millijoule levels in the 5 to 8 range. The need for higher millijoule levels may be related to the distortion of the beam and the effect of this distortion on the optical breakdown. Lysis of vitreous bands has been clinically reported by clinicians utilizing the YAG with resolution or improvement in clinical CME. Since the idealogy of CME is still controversial, the cause-and-effect result of utilizing the YAG will require further time and a more definitive answer. Although a little inflammation has been noted after lysis of the strands or adhesions, I have prophylactically put patients on topical steroids for one to two weeks following this lysis especially in cases of iris or vitreous strands (Figs. 68, 69).

Argon Laser Iridectomies

Argon laser iridectomies for glaucoma are widely used today in ophthalmology. This method requires skill and proper technique and can be difficult, particularly in light or blue irises due to the lack of pigmentation. The shock wave effect of the YAG laser has high potential in this area. One can see, even in light colored irises, snapping or rupturing of each strand of iris working down toward the pigmented layer. At this moment there are no available studies in the American literature on what happens to the lens capsule when going through the last part of the iris using the YAG. Therefore the use of any midzone iridectomy work in phakic patients should wait until that is proven safe in terms of rupture of the lens capsule.

Prior to that, the technique should be going into the periphery of the angle beyond the lens being careful of the angle of the beam and of the contact lens's being utilized so as not to get a perforation where it is not wanted. The use of the YAG in combination with an argon to get through the anterior iris and finish with the argon, and the use of the argon for coagulation and stretching effects prior to using the YAG is also recommended. In a few cases I have completed a sector iridectomy with the YAG to allow better visualization and later argon coagulation of ciliary processes. The effect of the YAG laser beam is quite striking in this type of case. Experimentally in rabbits and dogs a constricted pupil with a taut iris is easier to go through than a relaxed iris. Although it is possible experimentally in animals to rupture trabecular meshwork, clinical usefulness and effectiveness of this technique is still unknown. Since the nanosecond pulse appears to have little if any thermal effect, its use in trabeculoplasty does not appear indicated at this time (Fig. 70).

Vitreous Strands and Bands

Though vitreous strands are seen frequently, there are still many questions about the role that they play in retinal pathology—whether the cutting of them will make much difference in the treatment of vitreoretinal disease. There is no question, however, that vitreous bands, both pigmented and nonpigmented, can be readily lysed with the YAG laser either through a contact lens or a fundus lens when cutting vitreous strands and membranes. It is important again to keep the distortion of the beam to a minimum and therefore good quality optical lenses are also, again indicated. Certainly in a phakic patient one would have to be extremely careful of the proper focusing and keeping the energy levels down to minimize the size of the spark and the effects so as not to cause lenticular rupture or opacity. Forthcoming, but not available at this time, are good experimental studies detailing how close one can get to the retina in using the nanosecond pulse YAG laser. It certainly will be important to know if the safety zone is 1 mm or .5 mm or 2 mm. This of course will vary with the absorption through the vitreous and with the power level used. I recently had the opportunity to utilize varying YAG dosages on the retina and preretinally on a patient who was having an enucleation the next day for melanoma. We had varying doses at different levels on the retina and preretinally. Clinically, it appeared that there was little effect with the 1 and 2 millijoule pulses; but at the same time, I do not know what the actual level at the retina was in terms of absorption by the media and what may have been 1 millijoule on the readout may not have been much less at the retinal level. The tissue in this case is now being processed and will be reported later. Certainly if the YAG can be used safely on preretinal membrane pathology, this will become one of the important uses of this modality (Figs. 71, 72).

Summary

The Nd YAG pulsed Q-switched laser is a noninvasive surgical tool that allows lysis of membranes and bands in a variety of conditions. It appears to be safe and effective from its early reported usage. The complication rate appears to be low and the procedure appears to be particularly rewarding in comparison with invasive surgical procedures.

CONCLUSION

Pulsed YAG lasers, although they will not replace eye surgery, have opened a new wide field in ophthalmic therapy. They facilitate cataract ECCE, have made posterior capsulotomies safer and easier, and are very helpful in the treatment of both cataract surgery complications and glaucoma. They permit the sectioning of vitreous traction bands but are incapable of performing as well as a good vitrectome; they are also of little help in the treatment of proliferative retinopathy.

A basic principle must be understood: the faster a laser is pulsed, the safer it will be. New cutting lasers are in the experimental stage; an erbium laser is now being produced.

Alexandrite lasers (L 751-1 nanometer) may be pulsed in the range of the phemtosecond; because of its low average power, low peak power, and broad tunability, it seems to be extremely applicable in ophthalmic surgery. Alexandrite-laser-induced lesions on human tissue have been shown to be shallower and even more precisely limited than the picosecond one. This laser is still experimental, but is of great interest in the area of retinal work.

Some other possibilities may be offered with the already familiar pulsed YAG lasers, such as working through a mold with a totally computerized laser; radial keratotomy will possibly be achievable in a most perfect way.

We also could speak of the possibilities of the carbon dioxide lasers which provide good knives for both orbital and endocular surgery.

But the goal of this book was to provide a companion manual and to allow the ophthalmologists to become more familiar with this technique. We also hope that ophthalmologists will profit from six years of clinical experience in this field. Maybe we have reached one or two of these goals.

Councils to a Beginner

1. Focusing a YAG laser, especially a nanosecond laser, may be difficult; do not hesitate. *Use the laser beam coaxial,* and use a +45 to +60 diopters contact lens. The Abraham contact lens will be of perfect help.
2. Each time a posterior capsulotomy is to be performed behind a posterior chamber lens, even with the picolaser, one must do it through a +60 diopters contact lens. In doing so, you will very seldom pit the lens.
3. The combination argon laser and pulsed YAG laser works beautifully each time coagulation of vascularized tissue or blood vessels is required before YAG laser cutting.
4. Pulsed YAG lasers are efficient and not dangerous in trained hands. Ophthalmologists have to be properly trained and must know which are the indications, the limits, and the contraindications.

BIBLIOGRAPHY

I. GENERAL INFORMATION

1. AMAR, L, BRUMA, M, DESVIGNES, P, et al: Detection, d'ondes elastiques (ultrasonores) sur l'os occipital, induites par impulsions laser dans l'oeil d'un lapin. *CR Acad. Sci. Paris.* 259:3653, 1964.
2. ARON-ROSA, D, GRIESEMANN, JC: Pulsed Ultrarapid YAG Neodymium Laser. Section of vitreous strands and cyclitic membranes in the management of retinal detachment. Conferenza Internazionale sul distaco di retina, Rome, 29 Sep.–1 Oct. 1980.
3. ARON-ROSA, D, GRIESEMANN, JC, ARON, JJ: Applications ophtalmologiques des lasers neodymium YAG pulses—ouvertures preoperatoires des cristallins avant implant et des cataractes secondaires derriere implants cristalliniens. *J. Fr. Ophtalmol.* 4:61–66, 1981.
4. ARON-ROSA, D, GRIESEMANN, JC, JEANNEAU, E: Utilisation de lasers pulses en ophtalmologie. Application a la section des membranes intraoculaires. Congrès OPTO, Paris, 1980.
5. ARON-ROSA, D: Appareil de chirurgie ophtalmologique. Demande de Brevet Européen. No. de publication 0 007 256. No. de dépot: 79400370. 7 date de dépot: (07.06.78).
6. ARON-ROSA, D, ARON, JJ: Lasers in service of ophthalmology. *Impact.* 31:225–232, 1981.
7. BELKIN, M: Laser hazard. *J. Am. Intraocul. Implant Soc.* 6:334–336, 1980.
8. BIRNBAUM, G: *Optical Masers.* New York, Academic Press, 1964.
9. BLECKMANN, H, ZOEN, R: Akzidentelle laserkoagulation der Makula. Monatsbl Augenheilkd, 179:38–40, 1981.
10. CLAYMAN, HM: Lasers for ophthalmic surgery. *J. Am. Intraocul. Implant Soc.* 6:336–338, 1980.
11. COLEMAN, WF: Lasers—an introduction. *J. Chemic. Educ.* 59:   , 1982.
12. DANNHEIM, F, BASSOW, B: Zur laser trabeculopuncture. *Ophthalmologica.* 173:40–48, 1976.
13. DESVIGNES, P, AMAR, L, BRUMA, M, et al: Sur la formation d'ondes ultrasonores et formation de bulles dans le vitré d'un oeil humain par irradiation d'impulsion laser. *CR Acad. Sci. Paris.* 259:1588, 1964.
14. DIXON, JA, et al: Surgical applications of lasers. *Institute of Electrical and Electronics Engineers. Proceedings.* 70:   , 1982.
15. GEERAETS, WJ, BERRY, R: Ocular spectral characteristics as related to hazards from lasers and other light sources. *Am. J. Ophthalmol.* 66: 15–20, 1968.
16. HAM, WT, WILLIAMS, RC, MUELLER, HA, et al: Effects of laser radiation on the mammalian eye. *Trans. N.Y. Acad. Sci.* 28 (Ser. 11):517–526, 1966.
17. HU, C, BARNES, F: The thermal-chemical damage in biological material under laser irradiation. *IEEE Trans. Biomed. Eng.* BME-17:220–229, 1970.
18. KRAFF, M, PEYMAN, G, et al: Noninvasive casulecomy using a new pulsed infrared laser. *Am. Intraocular Implant Soc. J.* 8:239–247, 1982.
19. LENGYEL, BA: *Introduction to Laser Physics.* New York, John Wiley and Sons, 1966.
20. METCALF, R: Arthroscopy of the knee. *Orthop. Clin. No. Am.,* 1982.
21. McNAIR, J, FRAUNFELDER, FT, WILSON, RS, et al: Acute pressure changes and possible secondary tissue changes due to laser or xenon photocoagulation. *Am. J. Ophthalmol.* 77:13–18, 1974.
22. PRESSLEY, RJ: Principles of Nd:Yag Lasers. In *The Optical Industry and System Purchasing Directory,* ed. 26, 5 538-B 540, 1980.
23. PUTNEY, FJ: Carbon dioxide laser in otolaryngology. *Southern Medical Journal.* 72:1385–1386, 1979.
24. RIGGINS, J: Investigation of high power, pulsed neodymium YAG lasers for correcting opacities of the human eye. *Air Force Institute of Technology* AFIT/GEO/PH/82J-1, June 1982.
25. SAUNDERS, ML, et al: The use of the laser in neurological surgery. *Surg. Neurol.* 14:1–10, 1980.
26. SIEGMAN, AE: *An introduction to lasers and masers,* New York, McGraw-Hill, 1971.
27. SLINEY, D, WOLBARSHT, M: *Safety with lasers and other optical sources.* New York, Plenum Press, 1980.
28. SLINEY, D, VORPAHL, KW, WINBURN, DC: Environmental health hazards from high-powered, infrared laser devices. *Arch. Environ. Health.* 30: 174–179, 1975.
29. PEYMAN, GA: Intraocular photocoagulation with the argon-krypton laser. *Arch. Ophthalmol.* 93:2062–2064, 1980.
30. TOWNSEND, DE, MARKS, EJ: Cryosurgery and the CO2 laser. *Cancer* (July Suppl.), 1981.
31. YARIV, A: *Introduction to optical electronics.* New York, Holt Rinehart and Winston Inc., 1971.
32. YELLIN, AE: Gastric phototherapy and the argon-ion laser: a review. *Surg. Annu.* 13:185–203, 1981.

II. RESEARCH APPLICATIONS

1. BIRNGRUBER, R, HILLENKAMP, F, STEFANI, FH, et al: Q-switched ruby laser damage of the rabbit eye lens. *Adv. Ophthalmol.* 34:158–163, 1977.
2. CAMPBELL, Charles J, RITTLER, Catherine, et al: Ocular effects produced by experimental lasers. *Am. J. Ophthalmol.* 66:605–632, 1968.
3. CLEARY, SF: Laser pulses and the generation of acoustic transients in biological material. *In*

WOLBARSHT ML (ed.): Laser applications in medicine and biology. Vol. 3. New York, Plenum Press, 1977, pp. 175–219.

4. CLEARY, SF, HAMRICK, PE: Laser-induced acoustic transients in the mammalian eye. *J. Acoust. Soc. Am.* 46:1037–1044, 1969.
5. EARLE, KM, CARPENTER, S, ROESSMAN, U, et al: Central nervous system effects of laser radiation. *Fed. Proc. Fed. Am. Soc. Exp. Biol.* 24 (pt. 3):S129–S142, 1965.
6. FINE, S, KLEIN, E, NOWAK, W, et al: Interaction of laser radiation with biologic systems. 1. Studies on interaction with tissues. *Fed. Proc. Fed. Am. Soc. Exp. Biol.* 24 (pt. 3):35–47, 1965.
7. GOLDMAN, A, HAM, W, MUELLER, HA: Ocular damage thresholds and mechanisms for ultrashort pulse of both visible and infrared laser radiation in the rhesus monkey. *Exp. Eye Res.* 24:45–56, 1977.
8. GRIESEMANN, JC, DECROISETTE, M: Thermal wave propagation and shock formation in optical breakdown. *J. Appl. Phys.* 50:3915–3920, 1979.
9. HAM, WT, MUELLER, HA, GOLDMAN, A: Ocular hazard from picosecond pulses of Nd YAG Laser radiation. *Science.* 185:362, 1974.

III. PLASMA FORMATION

1. BATES, DR, KINGSTON, AE: Recombination and energy balance in a decaying plasma. *Proc. Roy. Soc. London.* 297A:10, 1964.
2. BATES, DR, KINGSTON, AE, MCWHIRTER: Recombinations between electrons and atomic ions. 1. Optically thin plasmas. *Proc. Roy. Soc. London.* 267A:155, 1962. 2. Optically thick plasmas. *Proc. Roy. Soc. London.* 270A:297, 1962.
3. BOCHER, JL, GRIESEMANN, JC, LOUIS-JACQUET, M, DECROISETTE, M: Self phase modulation in the breakdown of gases by ultrashort pulses. *Optics Communications.* 16:262, 1976.
4. BERNSTEIN, MJ, COMISAR, GG: X-ray production in laser heated plasma. *J. Appl. Physics.* 41:729, 1980.
5. CHAMPETIER, JL, MARIOGE, JP, METZ, J. de, MILLET, F, TERNEAUD, A: Utilisation de lentilles asphériques pour l'obtention d'éclairements élevés. *CR Acad. Sc. Paris Série B.* 266: 838, 1968.
6. COLIN, C, DURAND, Y, FLOUX, F, GUYOT, D, LANGER, P, VEYRIE, P: Laser produced plasmas from solid deuterium targets. *J. Appl. Physics.* 39:2991, 1968.
7. COLIN, C, DURAND, Y, FLOUX, F, GOYOT, D, LANGER, P: Etude expérimentale du plasma créé par laser sur cible cryogénique. *J. Phys.* 29 Suppl. 4—C3, 59, 1968.
8. DECROISETTE, M, GRIESEMANN, JC, LOUIS-JACQUET, M, ROCCHICCIOLI, JL, SALERES, A: Les processus d'absorption et leur rôle au cours d'une implosion par laser. Influence de la longueur d'onde. *Congrès National de Physique des Plasmas.* Paris, 6/10 Octobre 1976.
9. DECROISETTE, M, PIAR, G, FLOUX, F: Observation of induced Compton scattering in laser created plasma. *Phys. Letters.* 32A:249, 1970.
10. DECROISETTE, M, MEYER, B, PIAR, G: Observation de l'harmonique 2 dans un plasma créé par laser. *J. Phys. Suppl.* 32:119, 1971.
11. DRAWIN, HW: Collisional-radiative ionization and recombination coefficient for quasi-stationary homogeneous hydrogen and hydrogenic ion plasma. Rapport EUR CEA FC, Dph-PFC/SRFC, 1969.
12. ELTON, RC, ANDERSON, AD: Calculations useful in the determination of electron temperature from X-ray continuum radiation emitted from high temperature plasma. NRL Report 6541, 1967.
13. FLOUX, F, COGNARD, D, DENOEUD, LG, PIAR, G, PARISOT, D, BOBIN, JL, DELOBEAU, F, FAUQUIGNON, C: Nuclear fusion reactions in solid deuterium laser produced plasma. *Phys. Rev.* A1, 3:821, 1970.
14. GRIEM, HR, KOLB, AC, FAUST, WR: Bremsstrahlung from dense plasma. *Phys. Rev. Letters.* 7:281–282, 1959.
15. JAHODA, FC, LITTLE, EM, QUINN, WE, SAWYER, GA, STRATTON, TF: Continuum radiation in the X-ray and visible regions from a magnetically compressed plasma (Scylla). *Phys. Rev.* 119:843, 1960.
16. KRASYUK, JK, PASHININ, PP, PROKHOROV, AM: Experimental observation of stimulated Compton absorption of laser radiation in a spark. *ZETF Pis. Red.* 12:439, 5 Nov. 1970.
17. PEYRAUD, J: Théorie cinétique des plasmas, interaction matière-rayonnement. *J. Phys.* 29:306, 1968.
18. PEYRAUD, J: Théorie quantique de l'interaction plasma-rayonnement. *J. Phys.* 30:461, 1969.
19. PIAR, G, DECROISETTE, M: Influence des impuretés et de l'inhomogénéité d'un plasma sur la mesure de sa température électronique. J. QRST (A paraître).
20. SODHA, MS, SAWHNEY, BK, SAWHNEY, RL: Optimum harmonic generation in plasma. *J. Phys.* D, 3:377, 1970.
21. SOUBLIN, J, PIAR, G, BOCHER, JL, MEYNIAL, D: Application de la spectométrie de masse à l'analyse des cibles en deutérium servant aux expériences de création de plasma par laser. Communication privée, 1970.
22. SPITZER, L: Physics of fully ionized gases. Wiley Interscience Publishers, Inc., New York, 1962.
23. SUCKEWER, S: Excitation and ionization of atoms and ions in a non-thermal plasma. 1. Popu-

lations of excited levels. *J. Phys.* B, 3:380, 1970.
24. SUCKEWER, S: Excitation and ionization of atoms and ions in a non-thermal plasma. 2. Ionization equilibrium. *J. Phys.* B, 3:390, 1970.
25. TOMLINSON, R: Scattering and beam trapping in laser produced plasmas in gases, IEEE *J. Quant. Electr.* 5:591, 1969.
26. VEYRIE, P: Contribution à l'étude de l'ionisation et du chauffage des gaz par le rayonnement d'un laser déclenché. *J. Phys.* 29:33, 1968; 31:41, 1970.
27. VEYRIE, P, FLOUX, F: Breakdown wave, shock wave and radiation wave in laser created plasmas. AIAA Paper n° 68–678, AIAA Fluid and Plasma Dynamics Conferences, Los Angeles, California, June 24–26, 1968.

IV. CAPSULE DISCISSION

1. ARON-ROSA, D, GRIESEMANN, JC, ARON, JJ: Applications ophtalmologiques des lasers néodymiums YAG pulsé. Ouverture pré-opératoire des cristallins avant implant et des cataractes secondaires derrière implant cristallinien. *J. Fr. Ophtalmol.* 4:61–66, 1981.
2. ARON-ROSA, D, ARON, JJ, GRIESEMANN, M, et al: Use of neodymium laser to open the posterior capsule after lens implant surgery. A preliminary report. *J. Am. Intraocul. Implant Soc.* 6:352–354, 1980.
3. ARON-ROSA, D, GRIESEMANN, JC, ARON, JJ: Use of pulsed neodymium YAG laser (picosecond) to open the posterior capsule in traumatic cataract. A preliminary report. *Ophthalmic Surg.* 12:496–499, 1981.
4. ARON-ROSA, D: "Cold laser" for eye microsurgery described by French ophthalmologist. *Ophthalmology Times* 7, N° 8, June 15, 1982.
5. KEATES, R: "Interview: Neodymium-YAG lasers cut clear membranes". *Ophthalmology Times* Vol. 7, N° 6, June 1, 1982.
6. KRASNOV, MM: Laser phakopuncture in the treatment of soft cataracts. *Br. J. Ophthalmol.* 59:96–98, 1975.

V. LASER IRIDOTOMY/ TRABECULECTOMY AND GLAUCOMA

1. BASS, MS, CLEARY, CV, PERKINS, ES, et al: Single treatment laser iridotomy. *Br. J. Ophthalmol.* 63:29–30, 1979.
2. BONNEY, CH, GAASTERLAND, DE: Low-energy, Q-switched ruby laser iridectomies in Macaca Mulatta. *Invest. Ophthalmol. Vis. Sci.* 18:278–287, 1979.
3. COHN, HC, ARON-ROSA, D: YAG laser reopening of blocked trabeculectomy (in press). Amer. J. Ophthal.
4. FANKHAUSER, FW, ROUSSEL, P, STEFFEN, J, et al: Clinical studies on the efficiency of high power laser radiation upon some structures of the anterior segment of the eye. *Int. Ophthalmol.* 3:129–139, 1981.
5. FRAUNFELDER, FT, VIERNSTEIN, LJ: Intraocular pressure variation during xenon and ruby laser photocoagulation. *Am. J. Ophthalmol.* 71: 1261–1266, 1971.
6. HAUT, J, IMBERT, C, BERNY-MARTIN, F, et al: Experimental trabeculectomy with a monomode argon laser. *Ophthalmologica.* 176:121–132, 1978.
7. HOFFMAN, F, HARNISCH, JP: Schlemm's canal after trabeculoelectropuncture. *Albrecht Von Graefes Arch. Klin. Exp. Ophthalmol.* 203: 191–199, 1977.
8. KRASNOV, MM: Q-switched laser goniopuncture. *Arch. Ophthalmol.* 92:37–41, 1974.
9. KRASNOV, MM: Q-switched laser iridectomy and Q-switched laser goniopuncture. *Adv. Ophthalmol.* 34:192–196, 1977.
10. KRASNOV, MM: Laseropuncture of anterior chamber angle in glaucoma. *Am. J. Ophthalmol.* 75:674–678, 1973.
11. KRASNOV, MM, ZIANGIROVA, GG, AKOPYAN, VS, et al: Comparative evaluation of the damaging action of ruby apparatus. *Vestn. Ophthalmol.* 3:22–29, 1978.
12. MCNAIR, J, FRAUNFELDER, FT, WILSON, RS, et al: Acute pressure changes and possible secondary tissue changes due to laser or xenon photocoagulation. *Am. J. Ophthalmol.* 77:13–18, 1974.
13. POLLACK, IP, ALAN, AL: Iridotomies in cynomolgus monkeys using a Q-switched ruby laser. *Tr. Am. Ophthalmol. Soc.* 78:88–106, 1980.
14. POLLACK, IP: Laser iridotomy in the treatment of angle-closure glaucoma. *Ann. Ophthalmol.* 13: 549–550, 1981.
15. TICHO, U: Laser application to the angle structures in animals and in human glaucomatous eyes. *Adv. Ophthalmol.* 34:201–210, 1977.
16. TICHO, U, ZAUBERMANN, H: Argon laser application to the angle structures in the glaucomas. *Arch. Ophthalmol.* 94:61–64, 1976.
17. TICHO, U, MAHLER, J, SEKELES, E, et al: Low-energy laser trabeculotomies in primates. *Exp. Eye Res.* 33:11–18, 1981.
18. VAN DER ZYPEN, E, FANKHAUSER, F, BEBIE, H: On the effect of different laser energy sources upon the iris of the pigmented and the albino rabbit. *Int. Ophthal.* 1:30–48, 1978.
19. VAN DER ZYPEN, E, FANKHAUSER, F, BEBIE, H, et al: Changes in the ultrastructure of the iris after irradiation with intense light. *Adv. Ophthalmol.* 39:59–180, 1979.
20. VAN DER ZYPEN, E, FANKHAUSER, F: The

ultrastructural features of laser trabeculopuncture and cyclodialysis. *Ophthalmologica.* 179:189–200, 1979.
21. VAN DER ZYPEN, E, BEBIE, H, FANKHAUSER, F: Morphological studies about the efficiency of laser beams upon the structures of the angle of the anterior chamber. *Int. Ophthalmol.* 1:109–122, 1979.
22. WORTHEN, DM, WICKHAM, MG: Argon laser trabeculotomy in monkeys. *Trans. Am. Acad. Ophthalmol. Otolaryngol.* 78:371–375, 1974.
23. WORTHEN, DM, WICKHAM, MG: Laser trabeculectomy in monkeys. *Invest. Ophthalmol. Vis. Sci.* 12:707–711, 1973.

VI. RETINAL STUDIES AND VITREOUS SURGERY

1. ARON-ROSA, D, GRIESEMANN, JC, JEANNEAU, E: Chirurgie endoculaire au laser YAG néodymium pulsé ultrarapide. *Bull. Mem. Soc. Ophtal. Fr.* 93:73–75, 1981.
2. ARON-ROSA, D: Section des brides vitréennes au laser froid pulsé. *Conferenza Internazionale sul distaco di retina.* Rome 29 Sept.–10 Oct. 1980.
3. ARON-ROSA, D: Chirurgie des tractions vitréennes e *Congrès International d'Ophtalmologie.* San Francisco, 30 Oct.–3 Nov. 1982.
4. GIBBONS, WD, ALLEN, RG: Retina damage from suprathreshold Q-switch laser exposure. *Health Phys.* 35:461–469, 1978.
5. GOLDMAN, AL, HAM, WT, MUELLER, HA: Mechanisms of retinal damage resulting from the exposure of rhesus monkeys to ultrashort laser pulses. *Exp. Eye Res.* 21:457–469, 1975.
6. HAYES, L, WOLBARSHT, M: Thermal model for retinal damages induced by pulsed lasers. *Aerospace Med.* 39:474–480, 1968.
7. LANUM, J: The damaging effects of light on the retina. Empirical findings, theoretical and practical implications. *Surv. Ophthalmol.* 22:221–249, 1978.
8. LOTMAR, W, FANKHAUSER, F, ROULIER, A: Photocoagulation through the Goldman contact glass. *Arch. Ophthalmol.* 82:314–319, 1969.
9. MARSHALL, J, MELLERIO, J: Histology of retinal lesions produced with Q-switched lasers. *Exp. Eye Res.* 7:225–230, 1968.
10. MARSHALL, J: Thermal and mechanical mechanisms in laser damage to the retina. *Invest. Ophthalmol. Vis. Sci.* 9:97–115, 1970.
11. SCHMIDT, RE, TABOADA, J., BUTCHEE, WI: Suprathreshold retinal damage due to single 6 picosecond 1060 nm laser light pulses. *Aviat. Space Environ. Med.* 8:788–791, 1979.
12. TABOADA, J, GIBBONS, WD: Retinal tissue damage induced by single ultrashort 1060 nm laser light pulses. *Appl. Optics.* 17:2971–2973, 1978.
13. TARVIN, JA, SCHROEDER, RJ: Time-resolved spectrum of light reflected from laser-produced plasmas. *Phys. Rev. Letters.* 47:341–344, 1981.

VII. THE GERMAN EXPERIENCE

1. FANKHAUSER, F, VAN DER ZYPEN, E: Lasereffekte in der iris. Naumann GOH, Gloor B (ed): Wundheilung des Auges and ihre Komplikationen. Munchen. J.F. Bergmann Verlag, 1980, pp. 337–341.
2. FANKHAUSER, F, LOTMAR, W: Optischer Zusats sum Lichtkoagulator von Zeiss-Oberkochen fur das Arbeiten mit dem Spigelkontaktglas van Goldmann. Klin Monatsbl Augenheilkd 160: 218–220, 1972.
3. FANKHAUSER, F, LOTMAR, W, ROULIER, A: Vergleichende Behandlung de diabetische Retinopathie durch Photocoagulation mit dem Argon-Laser und der Xenon-Hochdrucklampe. *Albrecht von Graefes Arch Klin Exp Ophthalmol.* 183:334–347, 1972.
4. HAGER, J: Besondere mikrochirurgische Eingriffe. 2. Erste Erfahrungen mit dem Argon-Laser Gerat 800. Klin Monatsbl Augenheilkd. 162:437–450, 1973.
5. LUTZ, T, STEFFEM, J, FANKHAUSER, F: Laser zur Bethandlung von Erkrankungen des vorderen Augenabschnitters. *Klin Monatsbl* Augenheilkd 172:435, 1978.
6. RASSOW, B, WITSCHEL, B: Zur laser-trabeculopunctur. *Ophthalmologica* 170:362–369, 1975.
7. SPITZNAS, M, KREIGER AE: Experimentelle Argon laser Trabeculopunctur an Rhesusaffen. *Klin Monatsbl Augenheilkd-Trabeculopunctur* 165:165–170, 1974.
8. VAN DER ZYPEN E, FANKHAUSER F: Effeckte eines neuartigen Lasertyps auf fixiertes Gewebe der Kammerwinkelregion des Affenauges. *Klin Monatsbl Augenheilkd* 172:436–437, 1978.
9. VAN DER ZYPEN, E: Die Bedeutung de Alterveranderungen am Corpus ciliare des menschlichen Auges fur die Presbyopie und die Kammerwasserzirkulation. *Verk Anat Ges Jena* 69:665–671, 1975.
10. VAN DER ZYPEN, E: Uber die Bedeutung des Ziliarmuskels fur den Kammerwasserabfluss. Eine elektronenmikroskipische Studie. *Anat Anz* 130:245–252, 1972.
11. VAN DER ZYPEN E: Licht-und elektronenmikroskipische Untersuchungen uber den Bau and die Innervation des Ciliarmuskels bei Mensch und Affe (Cercopithecus aetiops). *Albrecht Von Graefes Arch Klin Exp Ophthalmol* 174:143–168n, 1967.

VIII. THE NANOSECOND YAG LASER

1. ARON-ROSA, D: 'Cold' laser for eye microsurgery described by French Ophthalmologist. *Ophthalmology Times* Vol. 7, No. 8, June 15, 1982.
2. ARON-ROSA, D, ARON, JJ, GRIESEMANN, M, et al: Use of neodymium laser to open the posterior capsule after lens implant surgery. A preliminary report. *J. Am. Intraocul. Implant Soc.* 6:352–354, 1980.
3. ARON-ROSA, D, GRIESSEMAN, J, ARON, J: Use of a pulsed neodymium YAG laser (picosecond) to open the posterior capsule in traumatic cataract: A preliminary report. *Ophthalmis Surg.* 12:496–499, 1981.
4. FANKHAUSER, FW: "Swiss Scientist Disputes French Laser Statements". *Ophthalmology Times* Vol. 7, No. 9, June 15, 1982.
5. FANKHAUSER, FW, ROUSSEL, P, STEFFEN, J, et al: Clinical studies on the efficiency of high power laser radiation upon some structures of the anterior segment of the eye. *Int. Ophthal.* 3:129–139, 1981.
6. VAN DER ZYPEN, E, FANKHAUSER, F, BEBIE, H: On the effects of different laser energy sources upon the iris of the pigmented and the albino rabbit. *Int. Ophthal.* 1:30–48, 1978.
7. VAN DER ZYPEN, E, FANKHAUSER, F, BEBIE, H, et al: Changes in the ultrastructure of the iris after irradiation with intense light. *Adv. Ophthalmol.* 39:59–180, 1979.
8. VAN DER ZYPEN, E, FANKHAUSER, F: The ultrastructural features of laser trabeculopuncture and cyclodialysis. *Ophthalmologica.* 179:189–200, 1979.

Danièle S. Aron-Rosa, M.D.

GLOSSARY

Beam Divergence

The full angle of the laser beam spread is usually measured in milliradian = 3.4 minutes of arc.

Bleaching

Dye bleaching phenomenon: When the light intensity increases, the more intense the light beam, the more transparent the dye becomes. When the dye radiation is allowed to reach the rear mirror (or reflector), a laser oscillation occurs.

Coherent Radiation

A collimated beam of monochromatic radiation whose wavefronts represent surfaces of constant phase. A light beam is said to be coherent when any point of the electric vector is related to that of any other point by a definite, continuous, sinusoidal function. One hundred percent coherence is unattainable. In practice, the radiation is spread over a very narrow waveband whose center is a wavelength, which has been stated.

Collimated Beam

A beam whose rays are "parallel," that is, the wavefront is plane with very low convergence or divergence.

Continuous Wave (cw)

The output of a laser, which is operated in a continuous rather than a pulsed mode.

An ANSI Z 136.1, a laser operating with a continuous output for a period greater than 0.25 s is regarded as a cw laser; in BS 4803: 1972 sustained radiation for periods greater than 0.1 s.

Controlled Area

An area where the occupancy and activity of those within is subject to control and supervision for the purpose of protection from radiation hazards.

Dye

Dye is a saturable absorber that ensures a passive Q-switch.

Usual dyes for yag lasers are Eastman Kodak solutions n° 9860, 9740, and 14015. The dye has to be diluted either in chlorobenzene, methylsulfoxide, or ethyl sulfide before being poured into the dye cell.

Duty Cycle

Ratio of "on" duration to total exposure duration for a repetitively pulsed laser.

Emergent Beam Diameter

The diameter of the laser beam (measured at 1/e peak irradiance points) at the exit aperture of the laser or other optical system, as expressed in millimeters.

Enclosed Laser Device

Any laser or laser system located within an enclosure that does not permit hazardous optical radiation emission from the enclosure.

Energy

The capacity for doing work. Energy content is commonly used to characterize the output from pulsed lasers and is generally expressed in joules.

Energy Surface Density

Energy per unit area. The intensity of electromagnetic radiation per unit area per pulse or radiant exposure, as expressed in J/m^2 or J/cm^2. This term is applied to pulsed lasers.

Exposure Limit (EL)

Maximal level of exposure to optical radiation at which no hazard is known to exist.

Free-Running

In a free-running laser both longitudinal and transverse mode will oscillate simultaneously without mode-to-mode amplitude in phase relationship.

To work in the picosecond range, one has to mode-lock the laser.

Hertz (HZ)

The unit that expresses the frequency of a periodic oscillation in cycles per second.

Intrabeam Viewing

The viewing condition whereby the eye is exposed to all or part of the laser beam and the eye is directed towards the laser.

Irradiance (at a Point of a Surface) (E)

Quotient of the radiant flux incident on an element of the surface containing the point, by the area of that element. Unit: watt per square centimeter ($W.cm^{-2}$).

Joule (J)

A unit of energy. One joule = one watt delivered for 1 second or water second.

Laser Action

The production of a collimated beam of coherent electromagnetic energy often characterized by a single wavelength, great intensity, and very low angular divergence.

Laser Region

That part of a electromagnetic spectrum in which laser action occurs. It includes some visible ultraviolet and part of the infrared. It extends roughly from 200 nm to 3.4×10^5 nm.

Lasing Medium

A material emitting coherent radiation by virtue of stimulated electronic or molecular transitions to lower energy levels.

Limiting Angular Substance (α_{min})

The apparent visual angle that separates intrabeam viewing from extended-source viewing.

Limiting Aperture

The maximum circular area over which radiance and radiant exposure can be averaged.

Lossy Medium

A medium that absorbs or scatters radiation passing through it.

Maser (Optical)

Old name for laser.

Maximum Permissible Energy Surface Density (EL)

The maximum value of energy surface density of a laser beam that (according to present medical knowledge) is not expected to cause bodily injury and that is detectable at any time during the life of the person who has been exposed to it.

Mode-Locked Laser (Phaselocked)

A laser that generates a train of pulses of very high frequency instead of producing a continuous output. This phenomenon has been observed with a long cavity, high-gain laser that has been run to obtain the maximum output power. Typically, a helium-neon system operating in this way might produce pulse widths of 2 ns at a rate of 75×10^6/s. A helium-neon system of pulse widths greater than 0.3 ns could have a peak mean power ratio of about 40. *Modelocking* or *phaselocking* means to force the oscillating mode to maintain a fixed relationship. The output as a function of time will vary in a well-defined manner. The oscillating modes are in phase.

Ultrashort pulses in the picosecond range are obtained for solid-state lasers (for example: YAG rod or alexandrite) by mode-locking.

Monomode

The divergence of the laser beam is reduced to a minimum. A laser is monomode when the whole energy delivery occurs along only one axis.

Nanosecond

10^{-9} second.

Open Installation

Any location, where lasers are used, that will be open to operating personnel during laser operation and may or may not specifically restrict entry to casuals.

Optically Pumped Laser

A laser in which the electrons are excited into an upper-energy state by the absorption of light from an auxilliary light source. This type of laser is usually pulsed, but cw systems are coming into use.

Optical Breakdown

Microexplosion generated when a very high power density of energy is concentrated on a very small surface. It is the ionization of the medium through an intense electric field caused by the optical beam. It generates acoustic and shock waves and looks like a small blue spark.

Oscillator

Laser oscillator; the source of light.

Plasma

Ionized gas reflective for = 1,066A°. Occurs in optical breakdown.

Plasma and Optical Breakdown Production in Working in the Picosecond Range

A picosecond yag delivers an output energy varying from three to six millijoules in a burst of seven spikes of 25 picoseconds each. A seven-nanosecond interval separates one spike from the other.

The energy of a spike varies from a very low initial peak power to a maximum and then decreases.

P_{exempt}

That output power of a laser for which no applicable EL for exposure of the eye may be expected, either with or without optical instruments.

Phemtosecond

10^{-15} sec.

Picosecond

10^{-12} seconds.

Power

Energy per unit time. The time rate at which energy is emitted, transferred, or received, usually expressed in watts (or in joules per second).

Power Surface Density

The average power of electromagnetic radiation per unit area or "irradiance" expressed in W/m^2. This term is applied to a cw laser.

PRF

Abbreviation for pulse-repetition frequency.

Pulse Duration

The duration of a laser pulse, usually measured as the time interval between the half-power points on the leading and trailing edges of the pulse.

Pulse Length

The duration of laser operation or exposure in seconds, milliseconds, microseconds, nanoseconds, or picoseconds.

Pulsed Laser

A laser that delivers its energy in the form of a single pulse or a train of pulses.

Q

Quality. When a maximum energy has been stored in the laser rod, a high Q condition is reestablished and the laser emits a giant pulse.

There are mechanical, electrooptical, or dye switches.

Q-Switched Laser

A laser that emits short (=30 ns), high-power pulses by utilizing a Q-switch.

Radiance, L, Active, Passive

Radiant flux or power output per unit solid angle per unit area ($W.sr^{-1}cm^{-2}$).

Radiant Energy, Q

Energy emitted, transferred, or received in the form of radiation. Unit : joule (J).

Radiant Exposure, H

Surface density of the radiant energy received. Unit : $J.cm^{-2}$ or J/m^2.

Radiant Flux (Φ), Radiant Power

Power emitted, transferred, or received in the form of radiation. Unit : watt (W).

Rayleigh Scattering

Scattering of radiation in the course of its passage through a medium containing particles that are small compared with the wavelength of the radiation.

Repetitively Pulsed Laser

A laser with multiple pulses of radiant energy occurring in a sequence or train.

Saturable Absorber

See dye.

Waist of the beam

The width of the beam at the focal point.

ILLUSTRATIONS

Preparation

The rabbits were sacrificed. By limbal injection the aqueous humor was exchanged for 2.5% glutaraldehyde in disodium/monosodium phosphate buffer. Corneas were trephined and kept in the buffer solution for four to six hours, then rinsed and conserved at 4° C till after fixation. The corneas were then cut under microscope into 1 mm^3 fragments, immersed in 2% tetraoxyde, then dehydrated and placed in Araldite.

Initially, light microscope studies were performed on the preparations after toluidine borate blue coloration to identify specific areas, then fine cuts were made, treated with uranyl-lead and examined under the electron microscope (E.M.). Human eyes were prepared in a similar way.

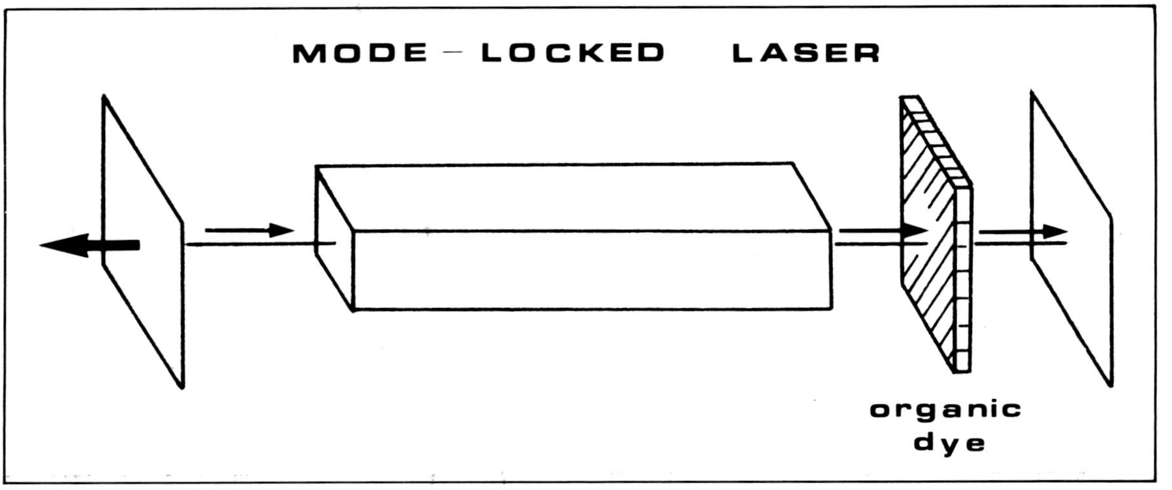

Fig. 1. A mode locked system (also called passive Q-switching) interposes an organic dye between the YAG crystal and the back mirror. The dye has the property of being bleached after a certain number of photons impinge upon it, but no light passes through till the critical point of bleaching occurs.

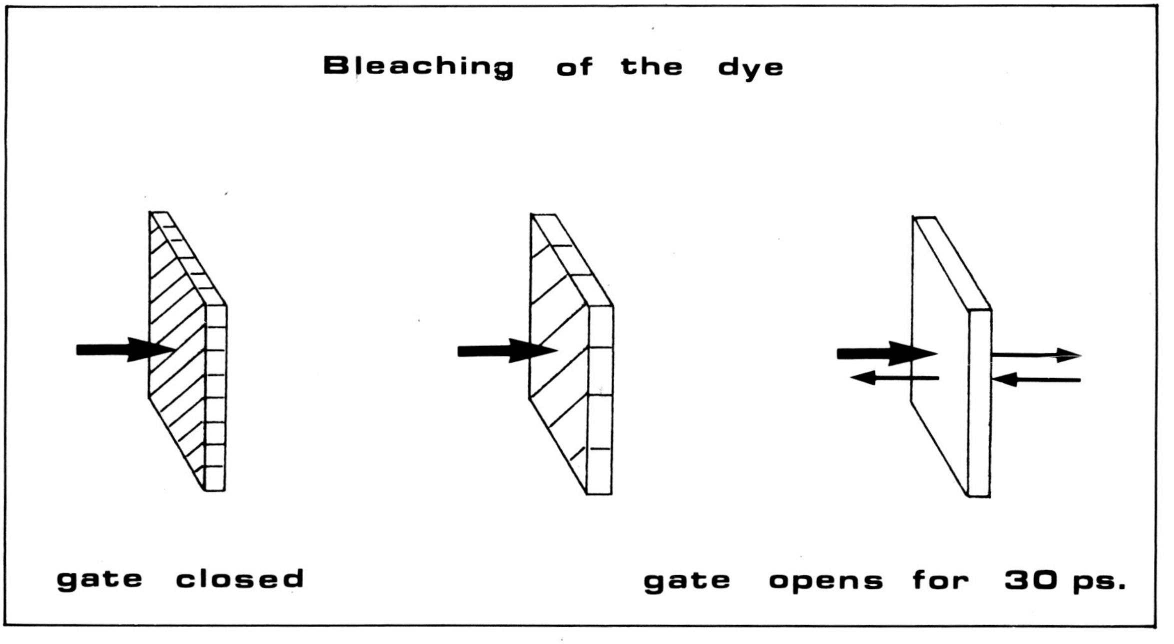

Fig. 2. Then the gate opens for several picoseconds and a series of picosecond pulses is produced for each strobe flash, with nanosecond intervals between pulses, as seen in Fig. 6.

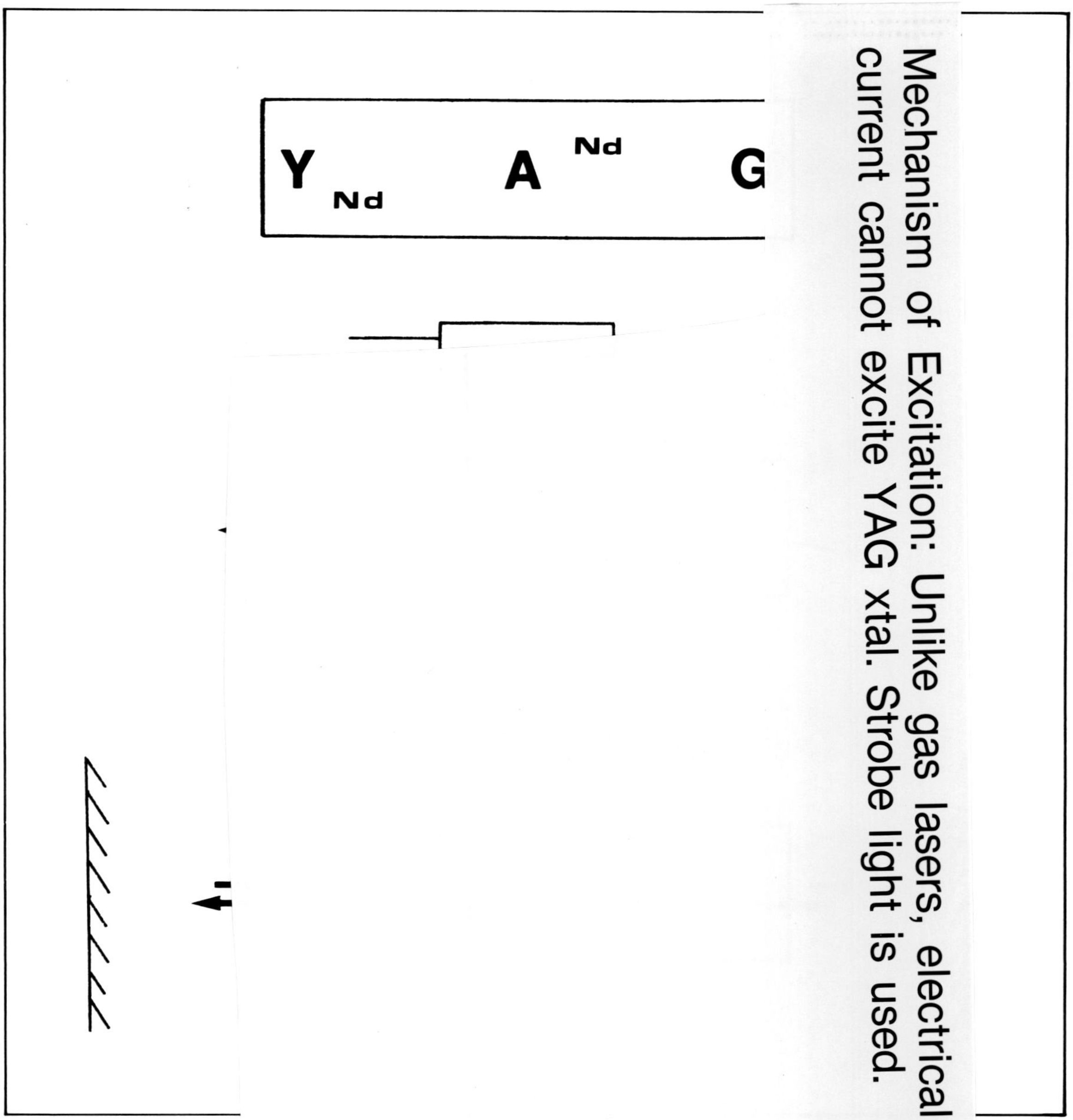

luminum
Neodym-
it is not
current
for gas
n is em-
off the
Neodymium atoms and Nd^{+3} is produced. These ions, in turn, then drop back to their unexcited state by emitting photons of light over a 10 millisec period (longer than the time of excitation.)

Figs. 4, 5. An active Q-switching laser system is demonstrated by replacing one fixed mirror of the laser cavity by a rotating prism. When the mirrored surface is not directly perpendicular to the cavity, no laser effect occurs. But, when the prism rotates into place, energy built up (that would otherwise be emitted more slowly) is suddenly released in a single grand nanosecond spike. This is called Q-switching since the Quality of the emission is being altered. Q-switching can also be achieved by an electro-optical shutter.

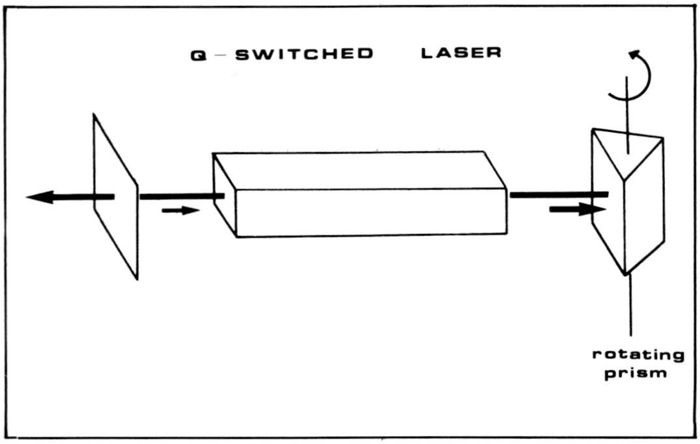

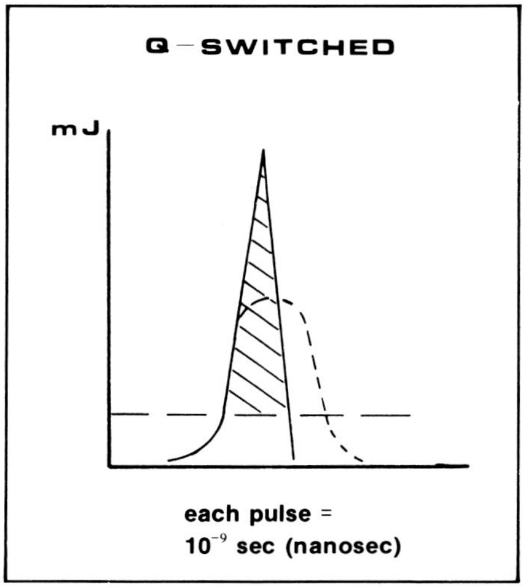

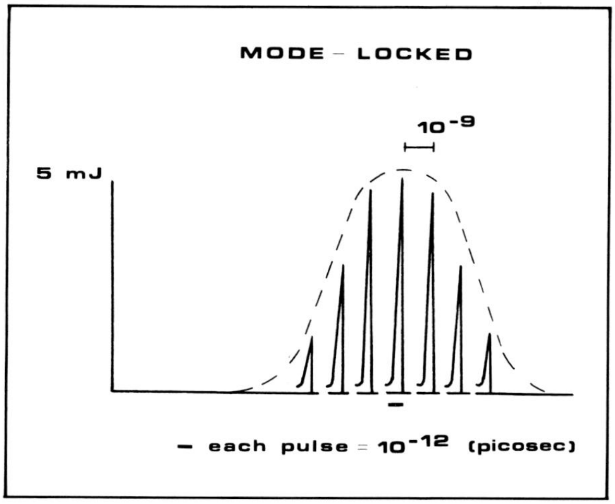

Fig. 6.

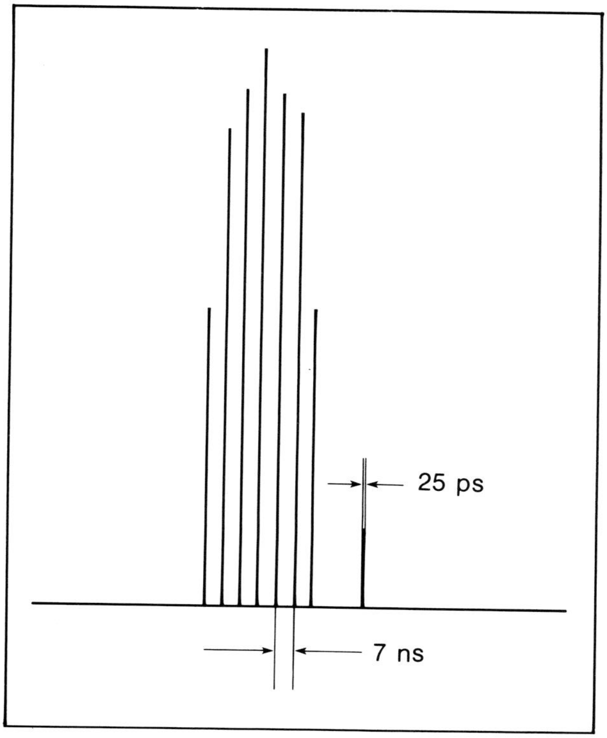

Fig. 7. Plasma and optical break down production working in the picosecond range. A picosecond YAG laser delivers an output energy varying from 3 to 6 millijoules in a burst of 7 spikes, of 25 to 30 picoseconds each; a 7 nanoseconds interval separates one spike from the other.

The energy of the spikes varies from very low initial peak power to a maximum, and then decreases as shown (eight to seven pulses in a Gaussian envelope).

Fig. 8. The picosecond monomode mode-locked Nd YAG laser mechanism of action.

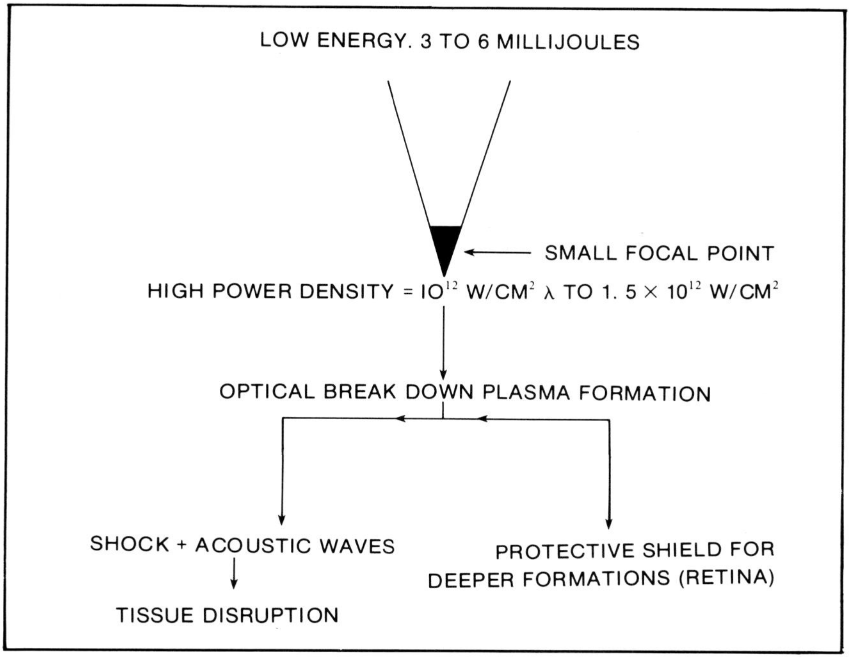

Fig. 9. The shock wave concept of YAG laser surgery: By delivering ultrashort pulses in the nano- to picosecond range, concentrated in a small area at the laser focus, enormous power density can be obtained ($\sim 10^{12}$ watts/cm^2). Optical breakdown takes place producing a centrifugal shock wave, and practically no heat is propagated. Mechanical disruption of the target tissue occurs independent of its pigmentation or chemical nature.

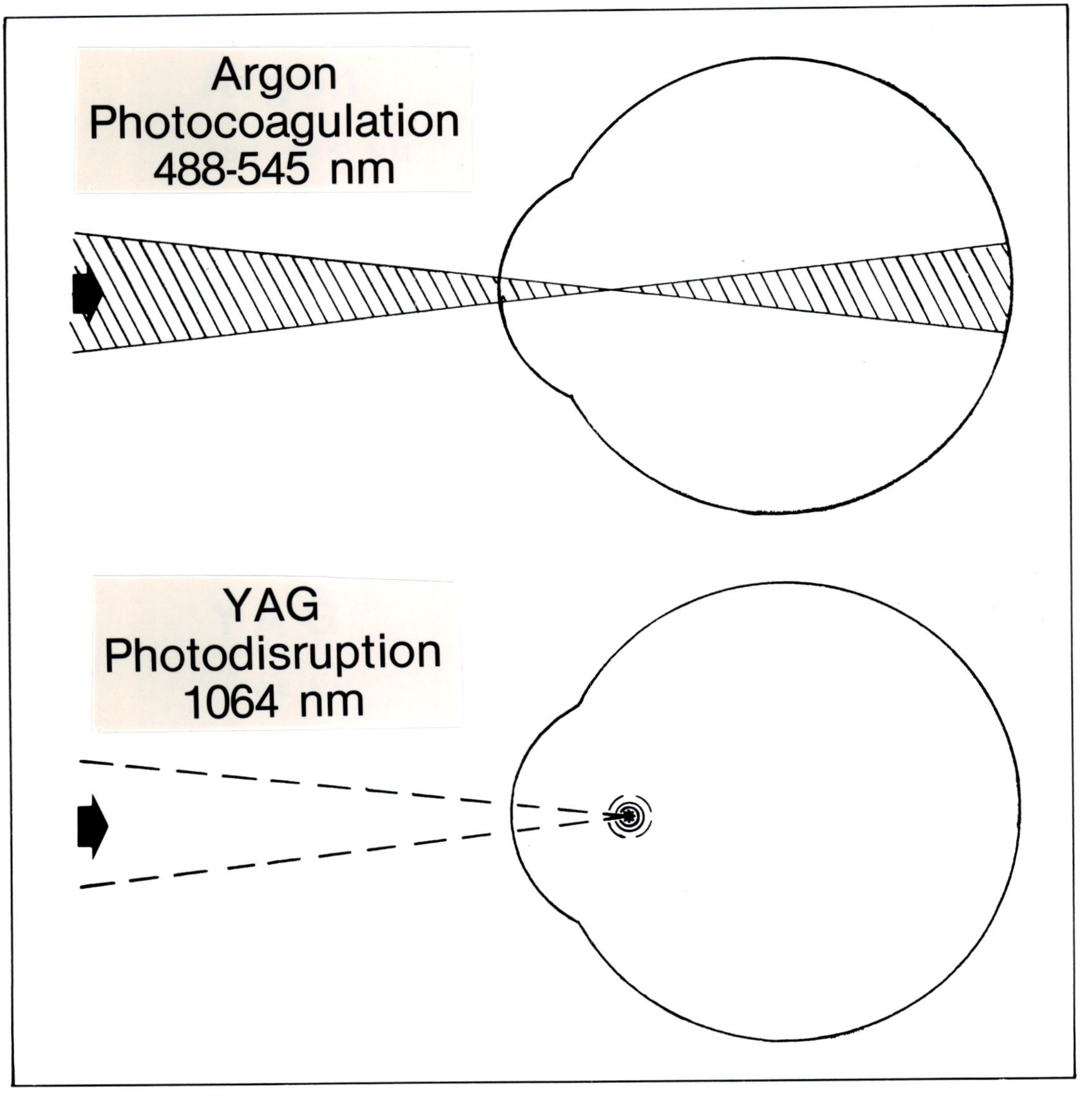

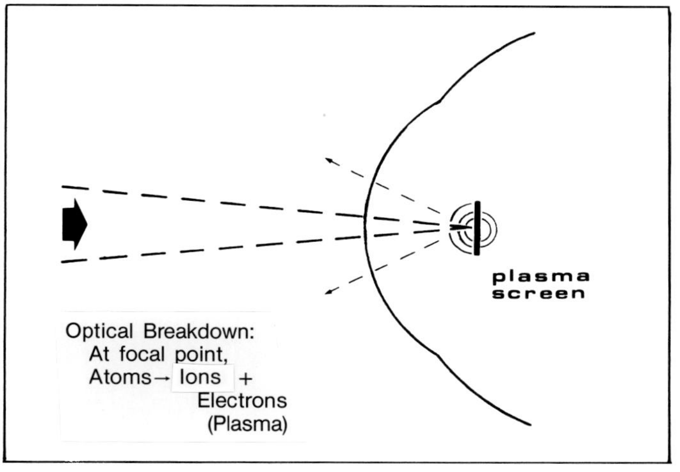

Fig. 10. The plasma screen concept: As optical breakdown develops, atoms at the area of laser focus are dissociated into ions and electrons forming a "gas" called plasma. Its high electron density (10^{21} e/cm^3) reflects back the 1064 mm wavelength of the YAG energy, affording relative protection of the retina when working in the anterior segment.

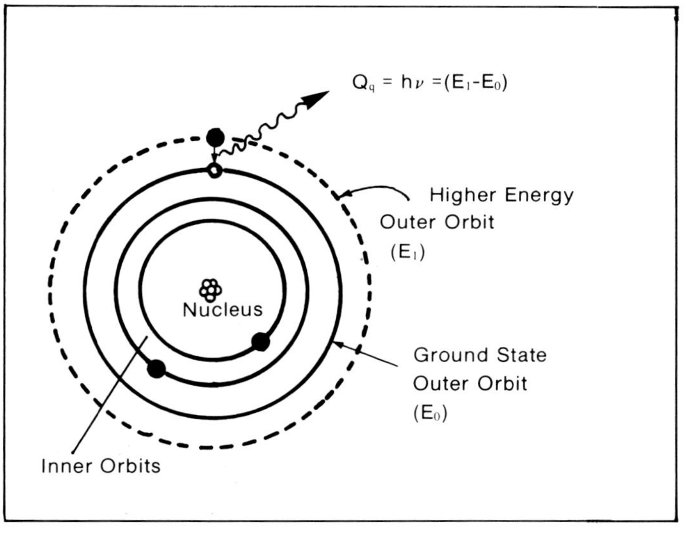

Fig. 11. Diagram of an excited atom. Transition of the outer electron from the higher energy orbit to the ground state orbit is accompanied by emission of a photon having energy equal to the difference between the energy levels of the two orbits.

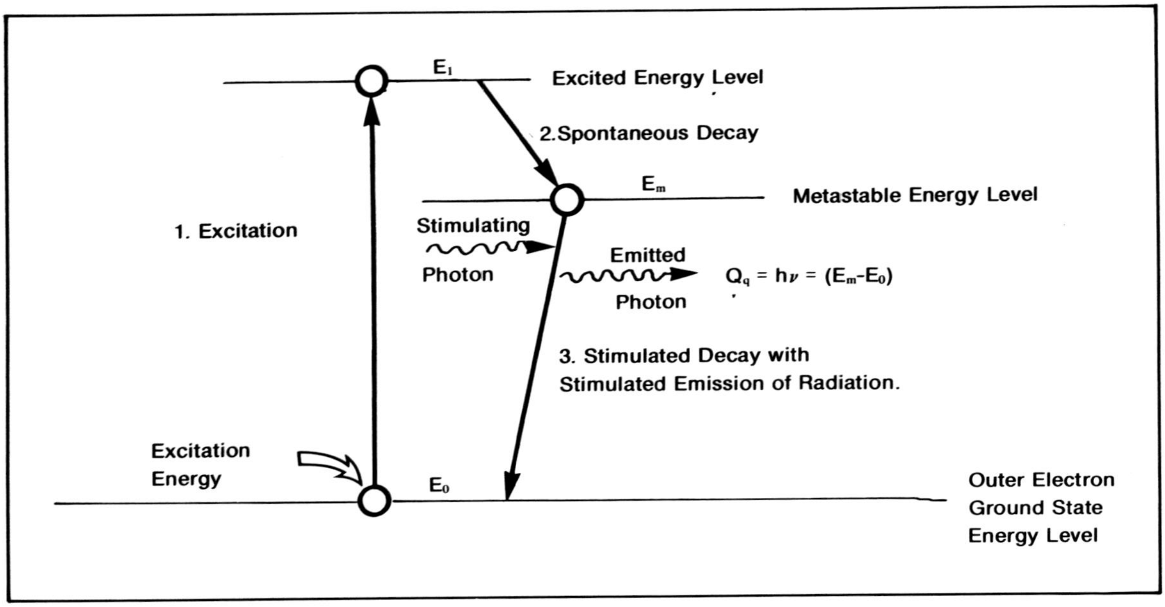
E1
Excited Energy Level
2.Spontaneous Decay
Em
Metastable Energy Level
1. Excitation
Stimulating
Photon
Emitted
Photon
Qq = hν = (Em-E0)
3. Stimulated Decay with
Stimulated Emission of Radiation.
Excitation
Energy
E0
Outer Electron
Ground State
Energy Level

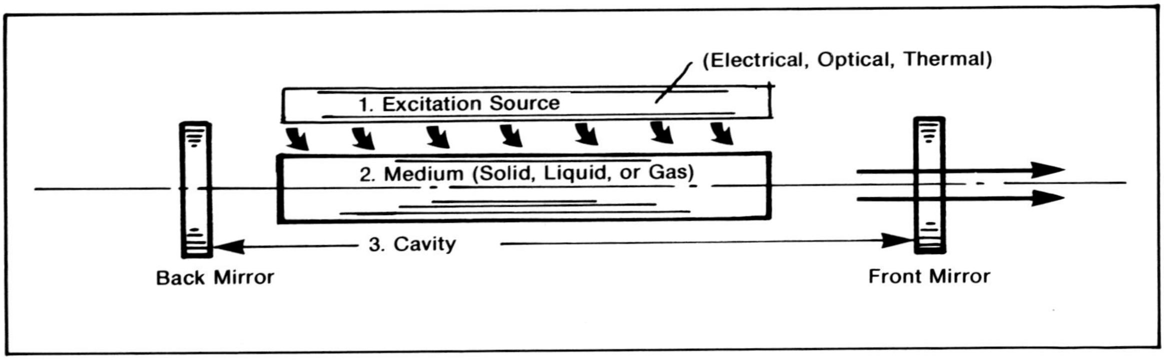
(Electrical, Optical, Thermal)
1. Excitation Source
2. Medium (Solid, Liquid, or Gas)
3. Cavity
Back Mirror
Front Mirror

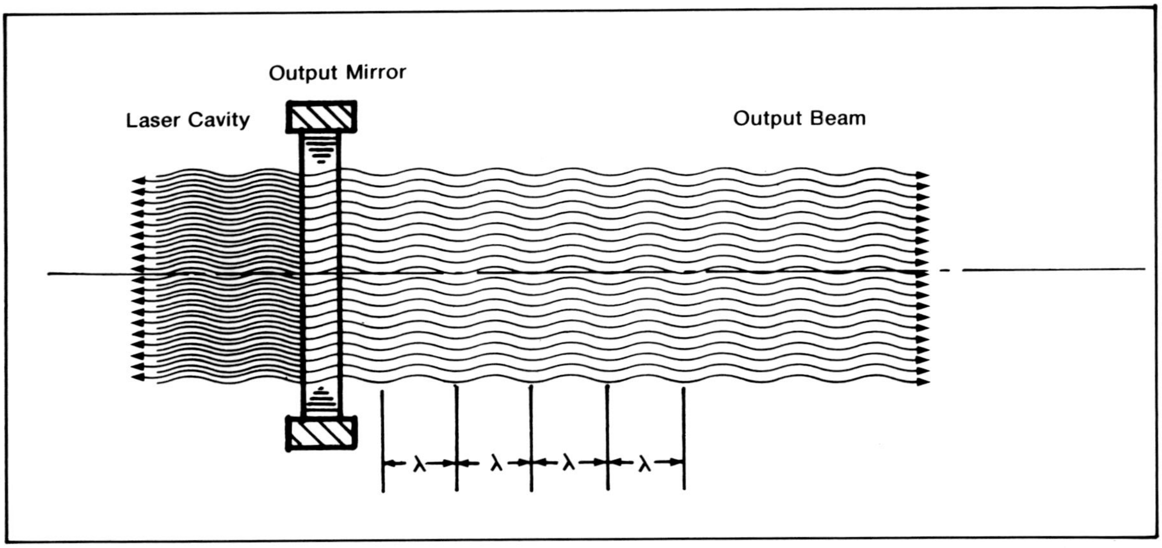
Output Mirror
Laser Cavity
Output Beam
λ
λ
λ
λ

Fig. 12. Three-level energy diagram. Upon entering the laser medium, exciting energy drives outer electrons to a higher energy orbit from which they decay spontaneously to a metastable, intermediate orbit. A stimulating photon of the proper energy induces decay back to the ground state with release of the stored energy in the form of a second photon.

Fig. 13. Three basic components of a laser. The excitation can be electric, optic, or thermal. The medium can be solid, liquid, or a gas. The cavity is bounded by mirrors. The back mirror is totally reflective; the front mirror is partly reflective and allows escape of part of the incident light from the cavity.

Fig. 14. Radiation leaves the laser cavity through the partly reflective output mirror with temporal and spatial coherence. The vibrations of the electromagnetic waves of the photons occur at the same time and at the same location. Distance between peaks is the wavelength, λ, of the light.

Fig. 15. Laser-induced anterior capsulotomy. One minute after laser application; plasma bubbles still present.

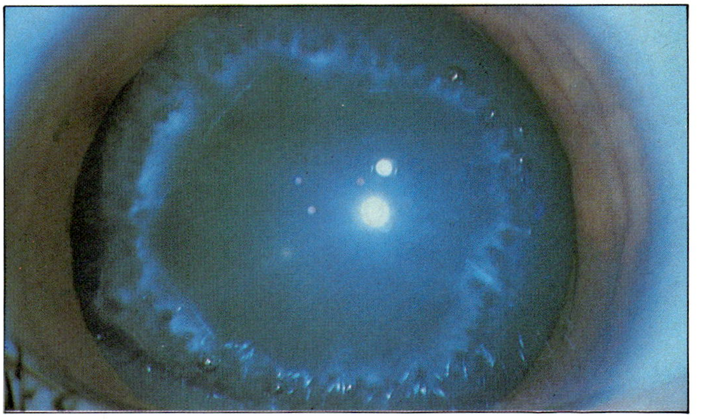

Fig. 16. Lens fragmentation. **A.** The lens was laser-softened before opening the anterior capsule; plasma bubbles trapped inside the nucleus. **B.** Plasma bubbles trapped inside the lens' nucleus.

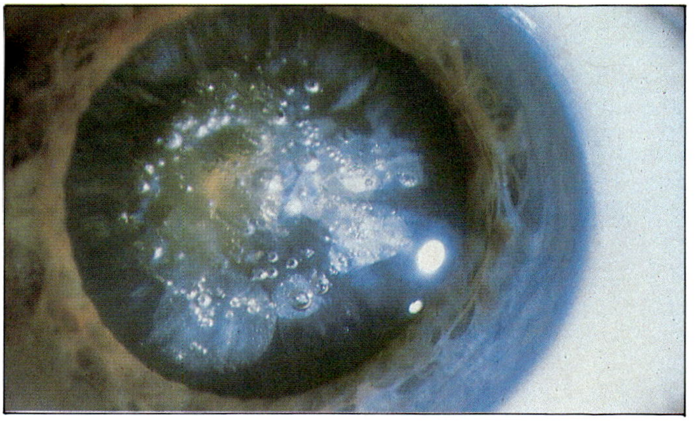

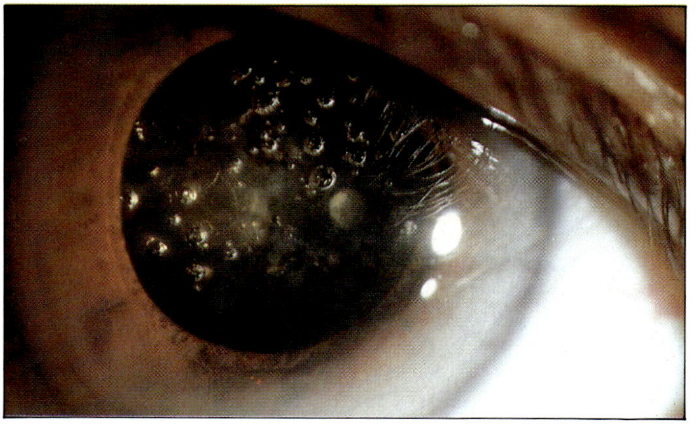

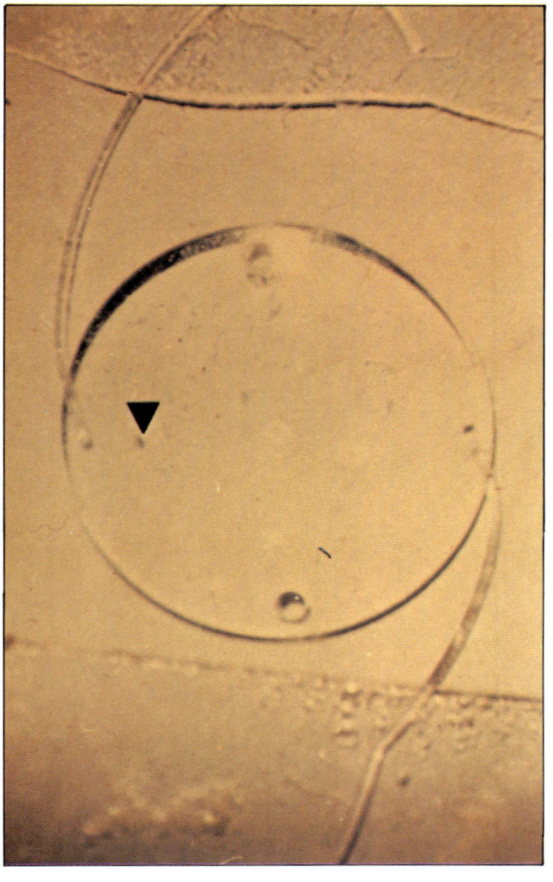

Fig. 17. A picosecond laser burst on a PCL (arrow).

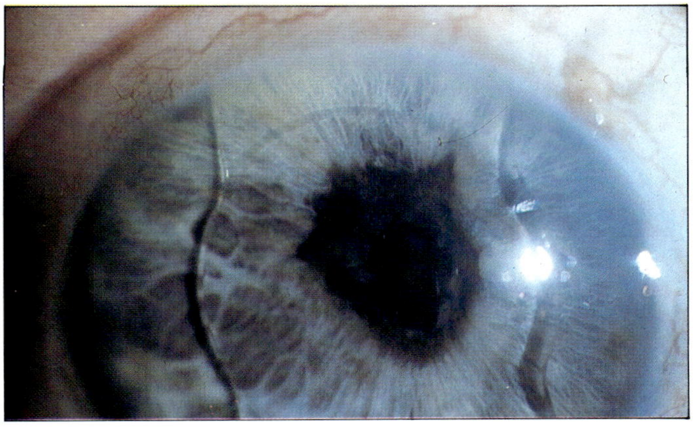

Fig. 18. Anterior chamber lens after laser-induced posterior capsulotomy. One shot.

Fig. 19. A. Before laser. **B.** After three laser shots.

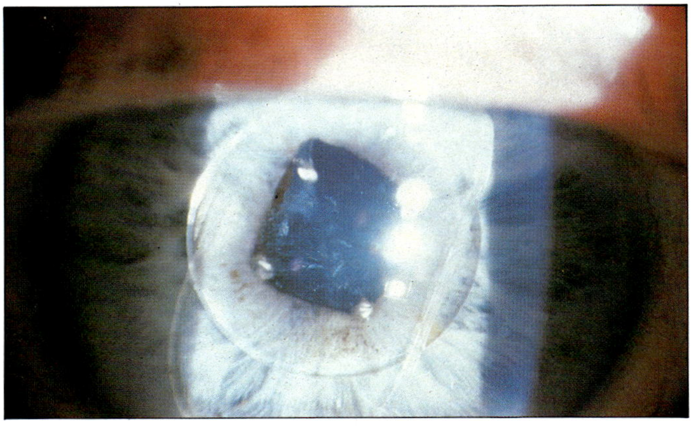

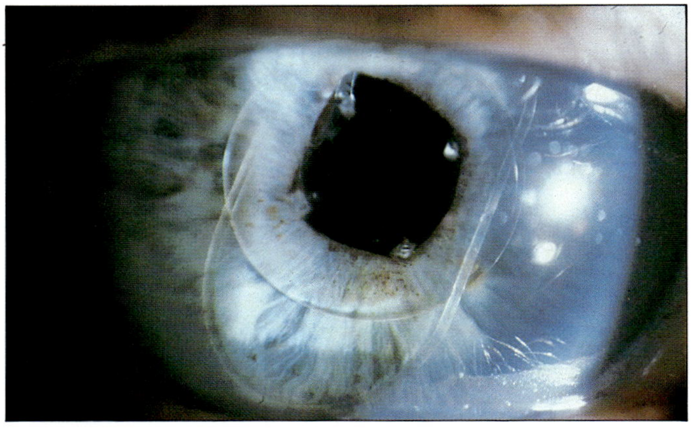

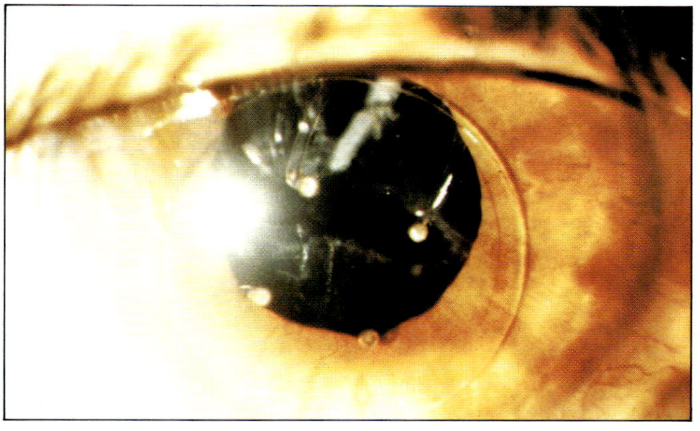

Fig. 20. Binkhorst 2 loops lens after laser-induced posterior capsulotomy. Four shots.

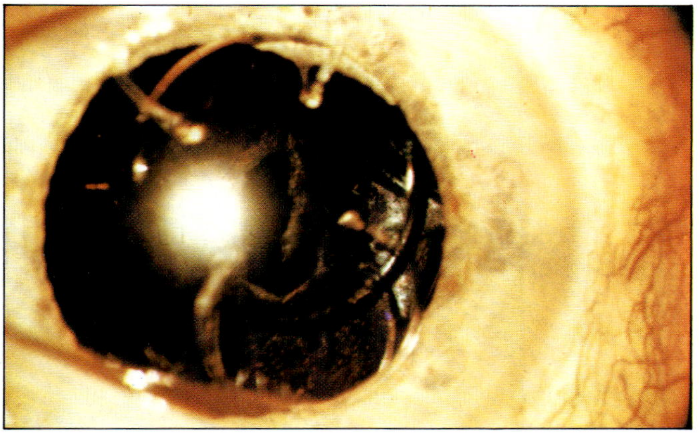

Fig. 21. Binkhorst 4 loops after laser-induced posterior capsulotomy. Two shots.

Fig. 22. Pseudophakos with opaque heavy posterior capsule and lens cortex. **A.** First laser burst (arrow). **B.** After ten laser bursts. **C.** At the end of the last (5th) session. Two pits on the IOL (arrows).

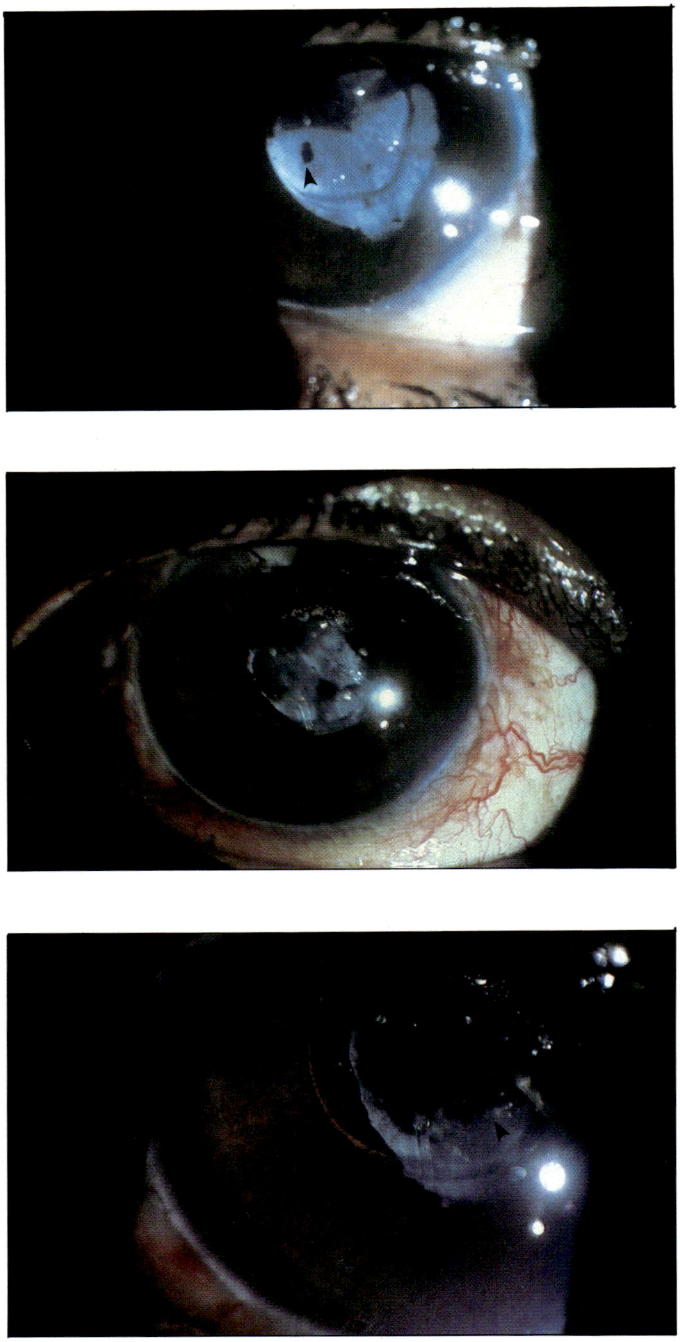

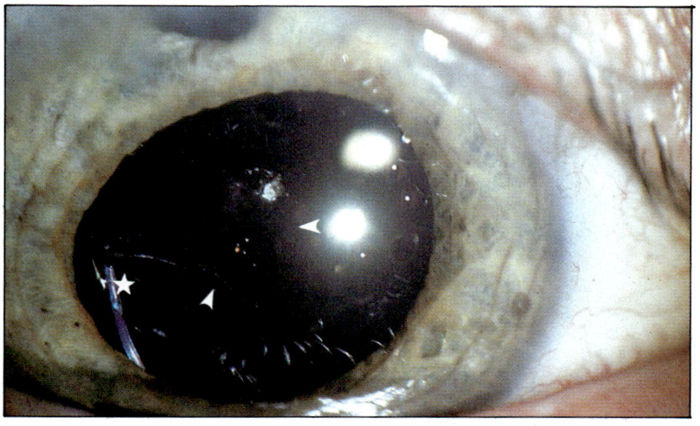

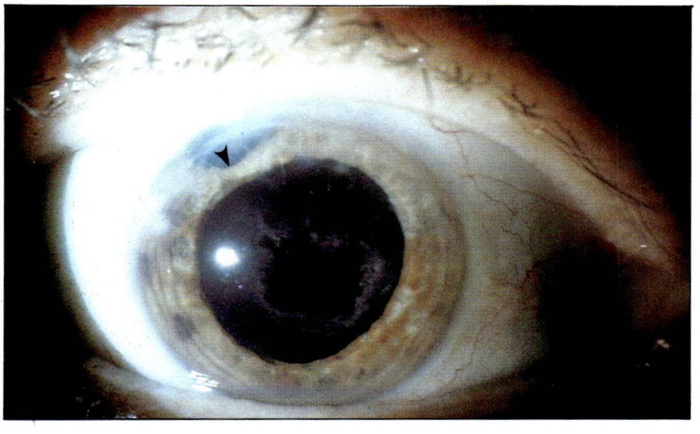

Fig. 23. Capsulotomy behind PCL. **A.** After one laser shot; note plasma bubble. IOL loop clearly visible. **B.** After six laser shots; square central capsulotomy. No pit visible on the IOL.

Fig. 24. A, B. Pseudopakic patient. Simcoe PCL after laser-induced posterior capsulotomy (ten shots). IOL pitted in three different places.

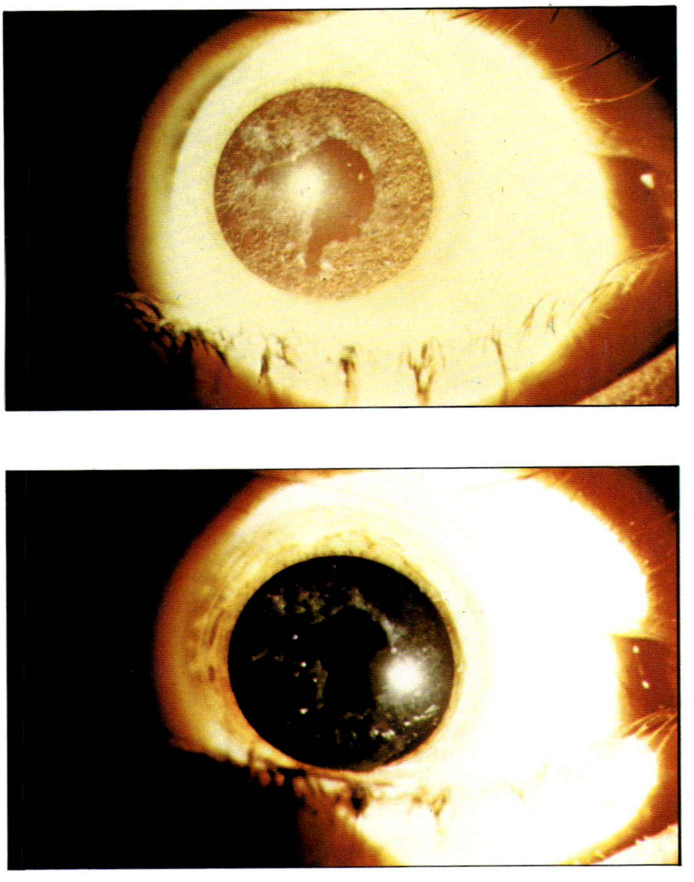

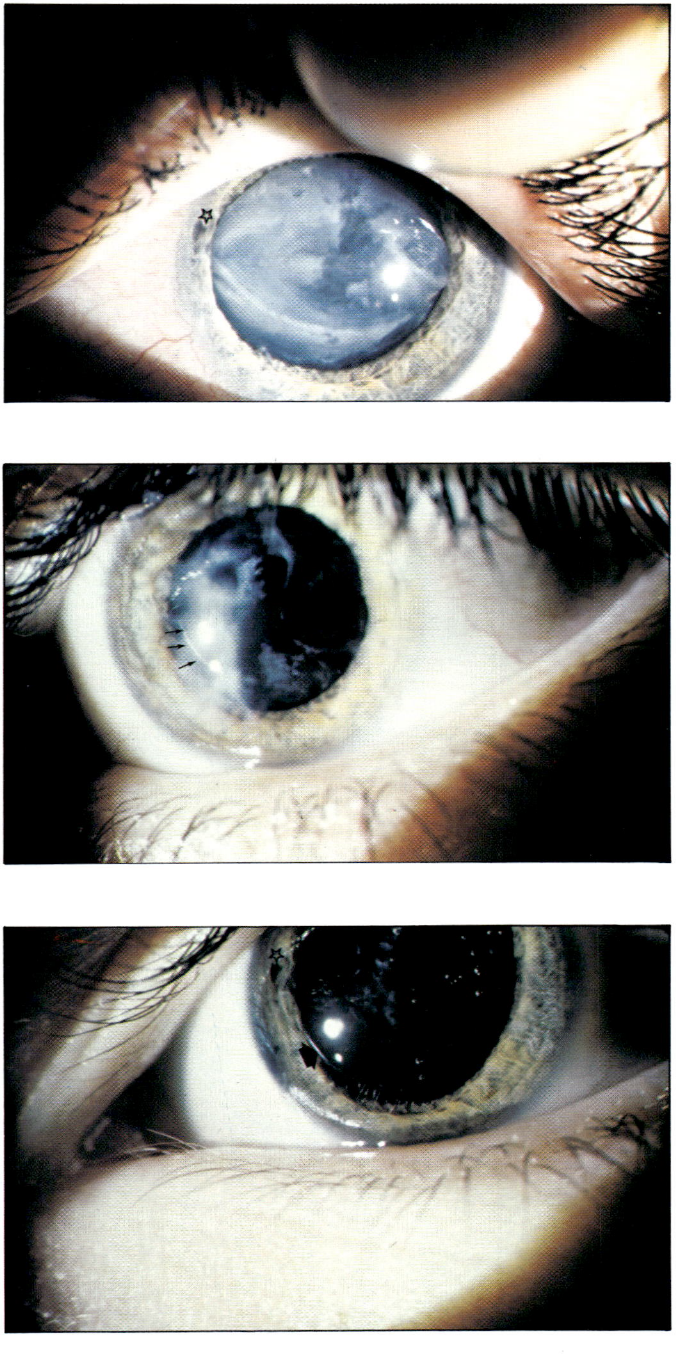

Fig. 25. Heavy cortex behind PCL. **A.** After the first laser session. Vertical opening of the remaining cortex. **B.** At the 4th session. Pseudophakos inferior border becomes visible (arrows). **C.** After the last laser application. Pupillary area has been cleared up; plasma bubbles still visible top right. Pseudophakos border visible (arrow).

Fig. 26. Picolaser cataract surgery in aphakic patients without IOL. Traumatic cataract: vertical capsulotomy. **A.** Before picolaser treatment. **B.** After 40 shots and one session.

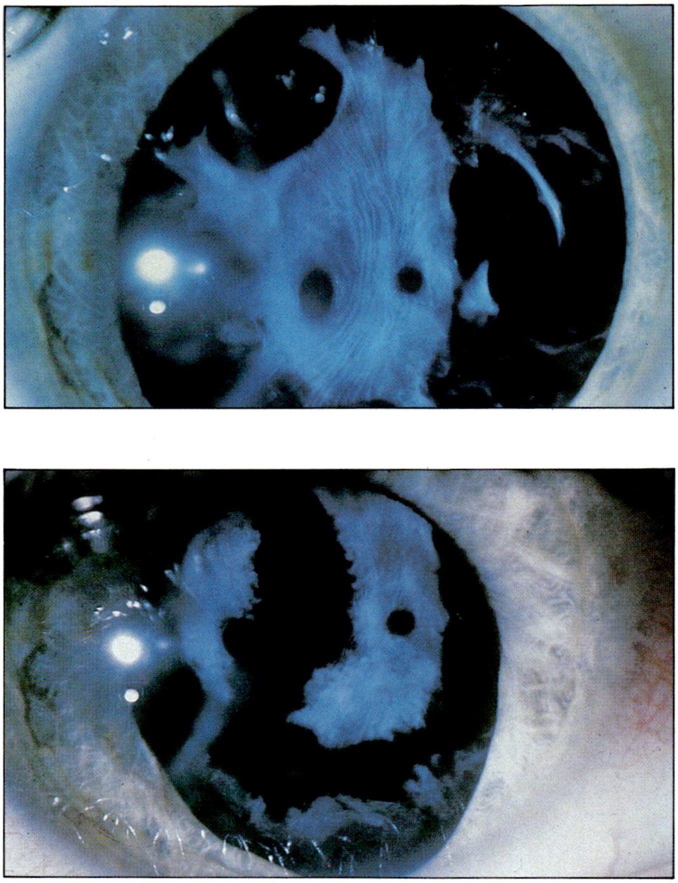

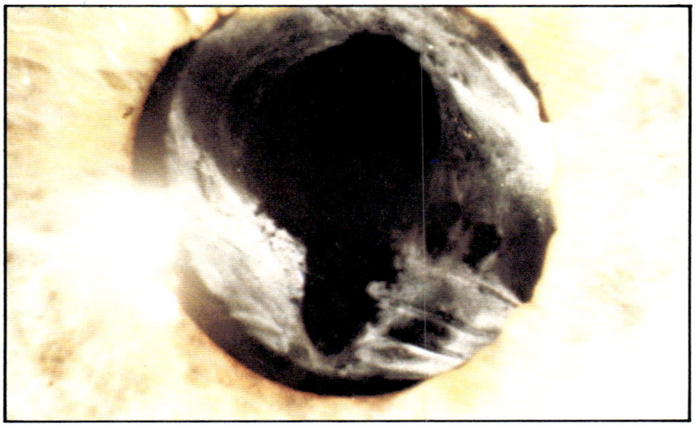

Fig. 27. Opacified capsule after incomplete extracapsular surgery (no IOL). The laser bursts have been applied perpendicular to the capsular fibers' traction. Wide opening of the posterior capsule was obtained after eight vertical bursts.

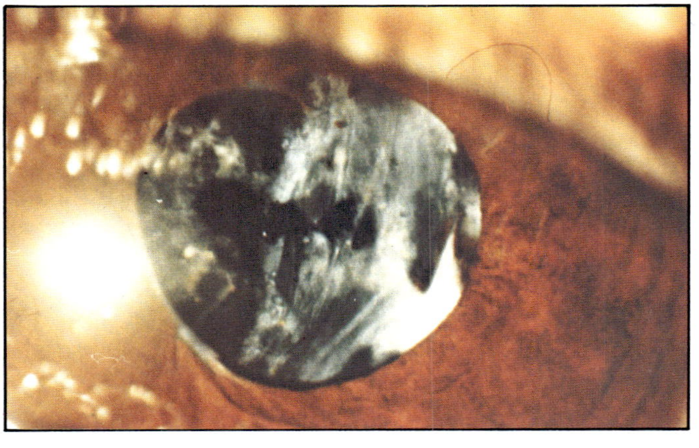

Fig. 28. Opacified capsule after incomplete extracapsular surgery (no IOL). The laser bursts have been applied perpendicular to the capsular fibers' traction. Heavier lens material. The horizontal opening after fifteen shots is still incomplete.

Fig. 29. Eventful cataract surgery. **A.** Before laser application. **B.** At the second session note iris lens synechiae has been released. **C.** At the fifth session four weeks later.

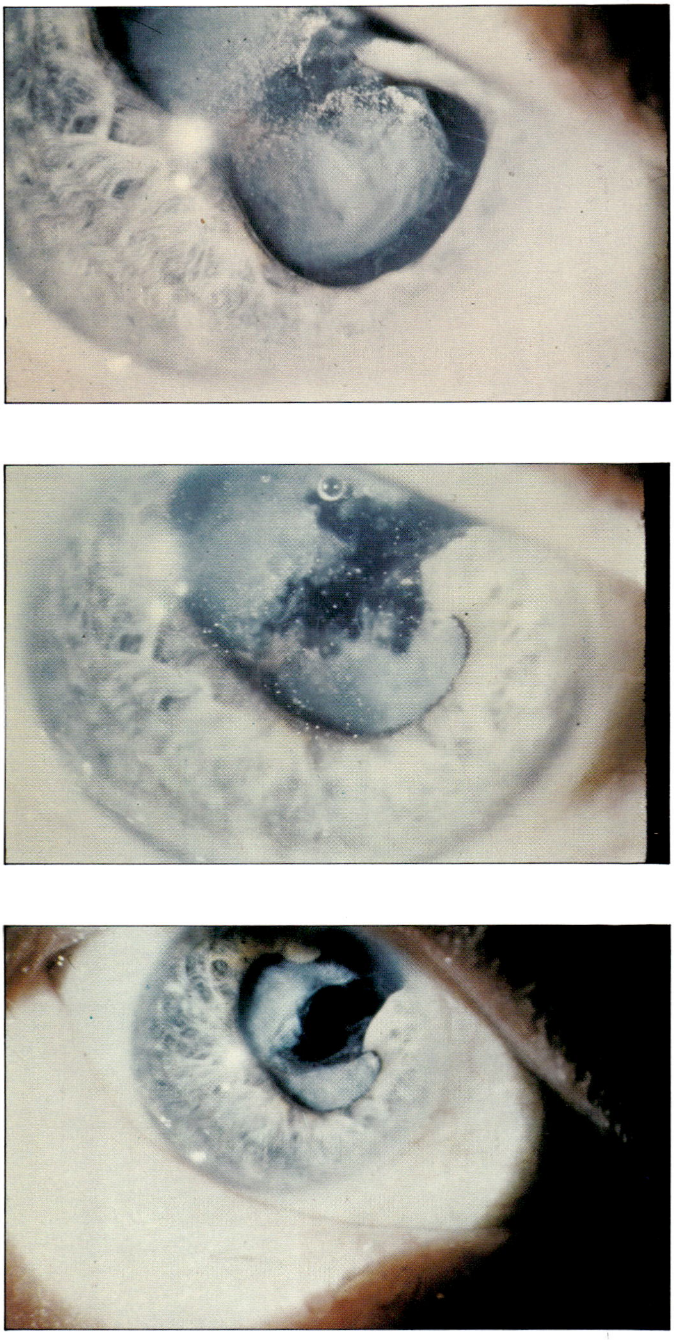

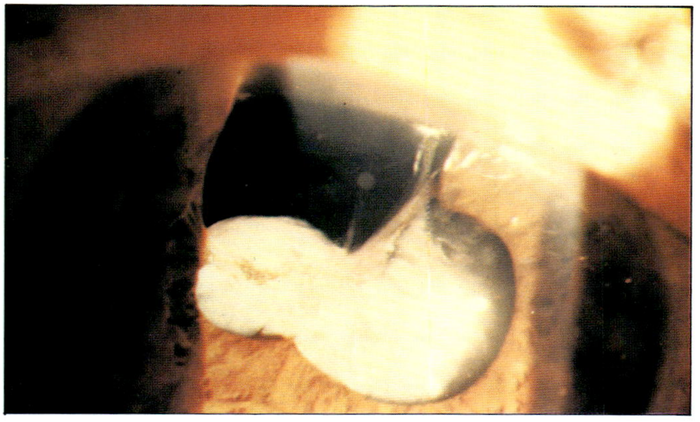

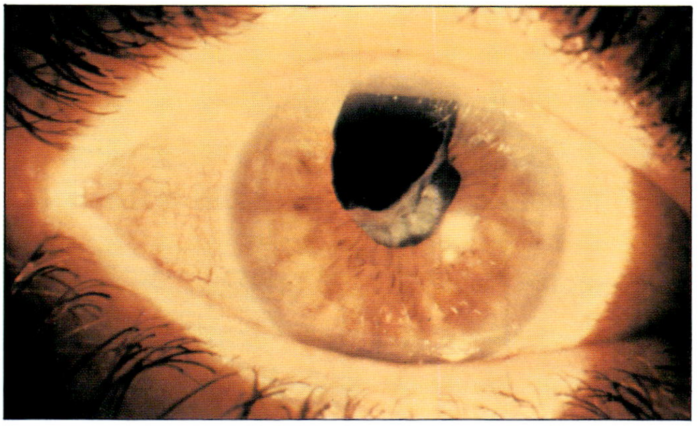

Fig. 30. Heavy lens material remaining in an aphakic patient without IOL. **A.** Before laser application. **B.** At the third session two weeks later.

Fig. 31A. Total pupillary adhesion to lens material before laser treatment; vision reduced to light perception.

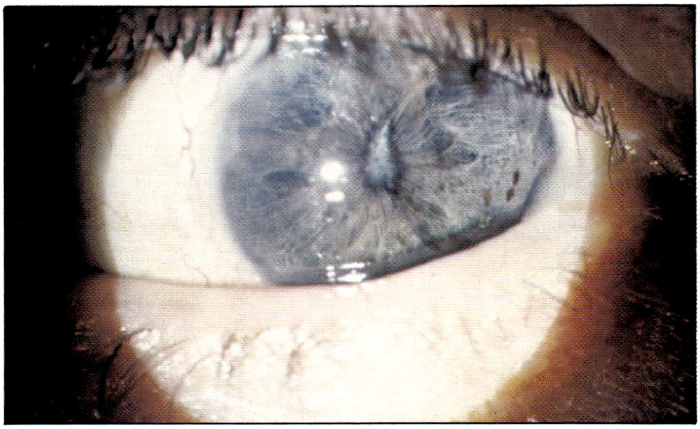

Fig. 31B. After the last laser session (ten sessions) at the seventh week; vision 20/25 with aphakic glasses.

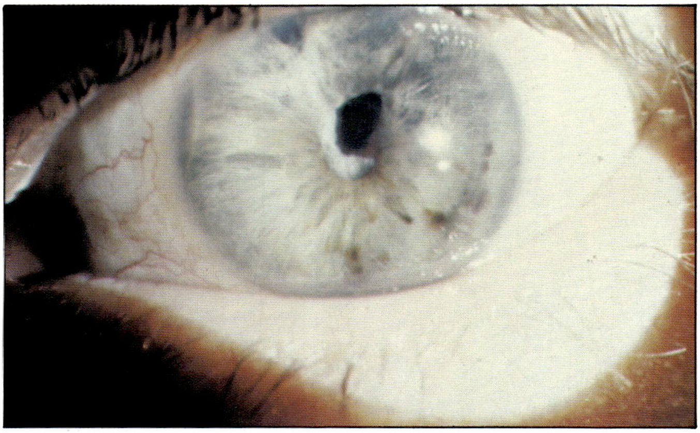

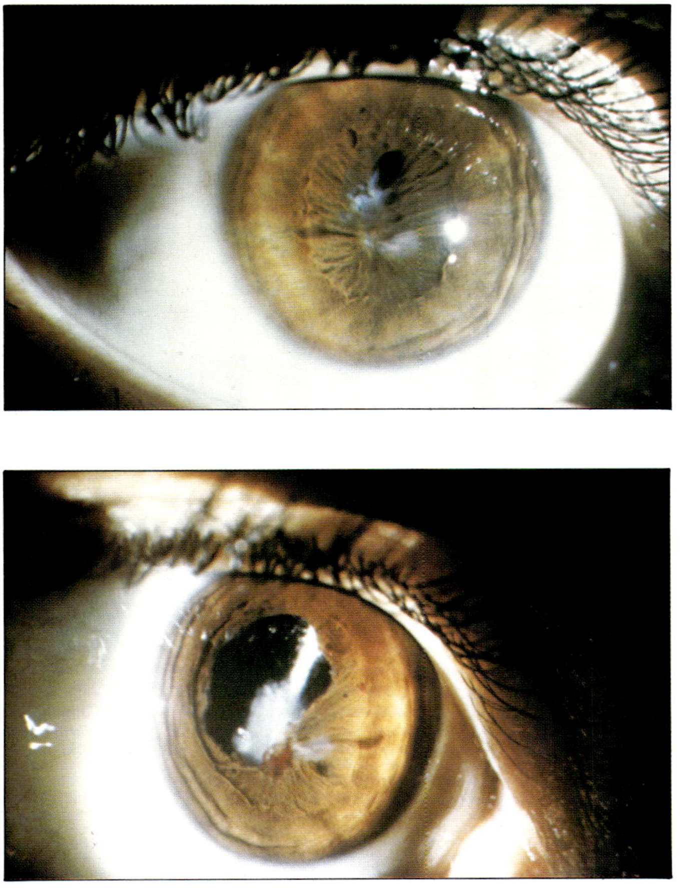

Fig. 32. Aphakic patient without IOL irido vitreous adhesions. IOP normal, **A.** Before laser treatment. **B.** After 3 laser bursts, the pupil has well opened. Note slight bleeding on the inferior iris border.

Fig. 33. Pseudophakic patient. **A.** Wavy irido pseudophakos adhesions and cyclitic membrane 18 months after surgery. Quiet eye IOP = 14 mm Hg previous to laser treatment. **B.** After 5 laser shots, bubbles trapped behind IOL; slight bleeding of the iris border. Central efficient perforation of the membrane half-hidden behind a bubble.

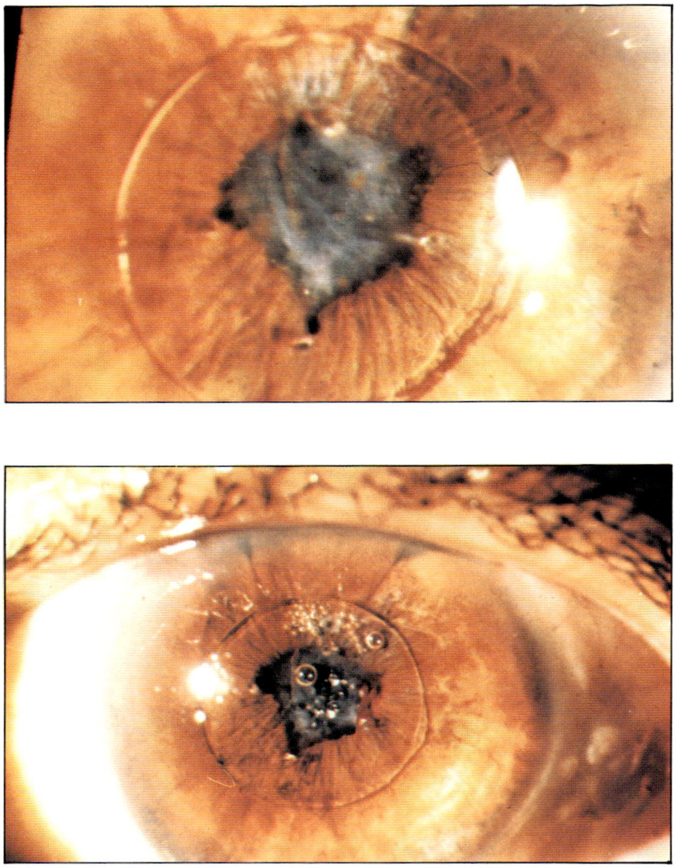

Fig. 34. Pupillary block in aphakic patient: increased IOP 38 mm Hg; hazy cornea; iris bombé. After two laser bursts, anterior chamber is deeper. A slight bleeding is visible at the site of the second shot which hit a blood vessel. IOP returned to normal at the 6th hour. New recurrences after 2 years' follow-up.

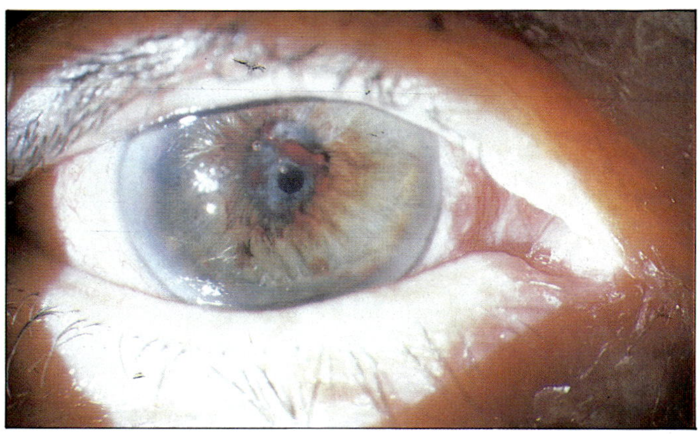

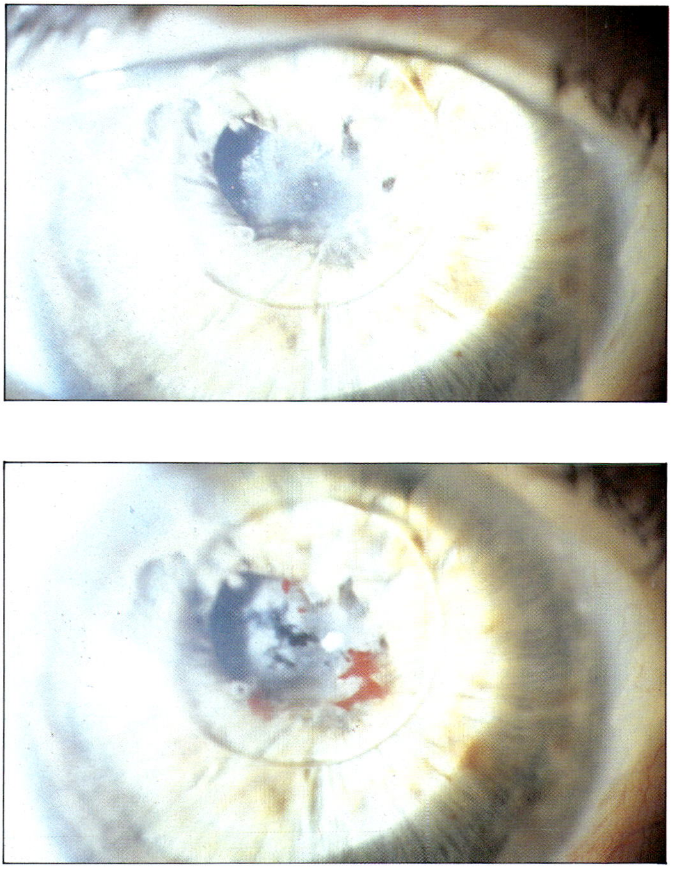

Fig. 35. Pseudophakic patients. Pupillary block increased IOP. **A.** Before laser application: flat anterior chamber, hazy cornea. IOP = 42 mm Hg. **B.** After the first laser session, anterior chamber is deeper. Note slight bleeding caused by laser shots on the vascularized iris.

Fig. 36. Laser disruption of inflammatory membranes in aphakic patient. **A.** After 52 laser shots. **B.** After 2 more laser bursts at the site of traction membrane (arrows). The pupil is wide open and the iris has gone back to a normal position.

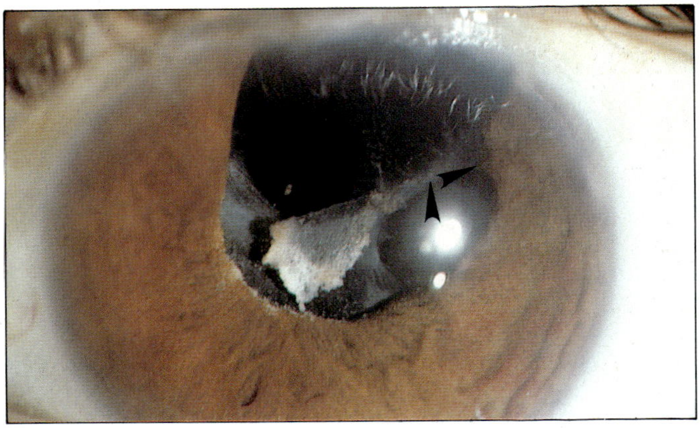

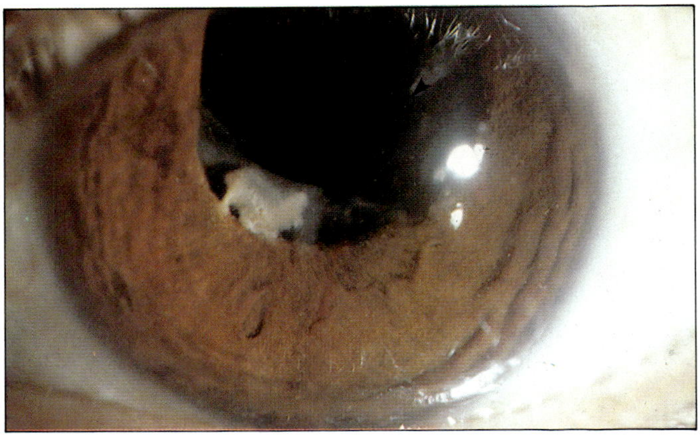

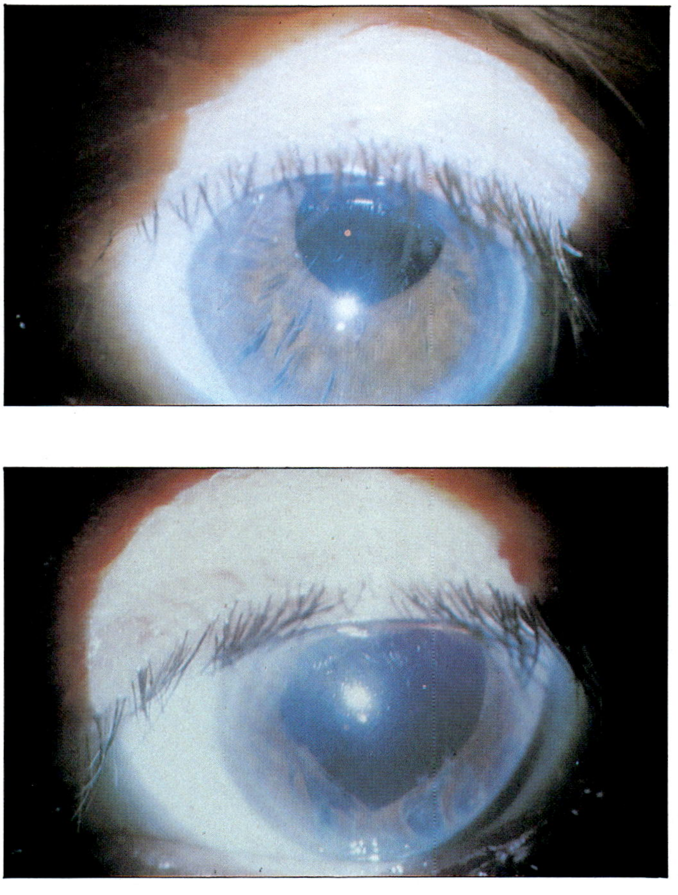

Fig. 37. Aphakic patient. No IOL; pupillary ascension. **A.** Before laser treatment, iris very tense; no abnormal vascularization was noted. **B.** After picolaser application. No bleeding visible. 15 laser shots were quite sufficient for a good opening.

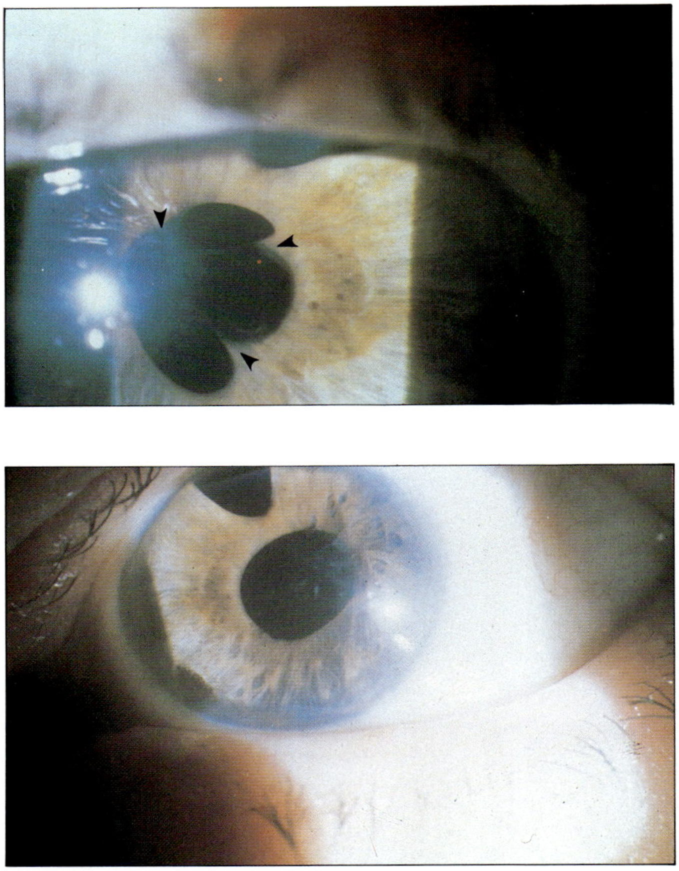

Fig. 38. Clover pupil, traction bands connecting the posterior pole to the iris, CME present, vision 20/400. **A.** Before laser treatment. **B.** After 3 picosecond bursts located near the iris border; pupil has become round and regular; 6 weeks later vision improved and remained improved at 20/35; CME better but still present at flourescein angiography.

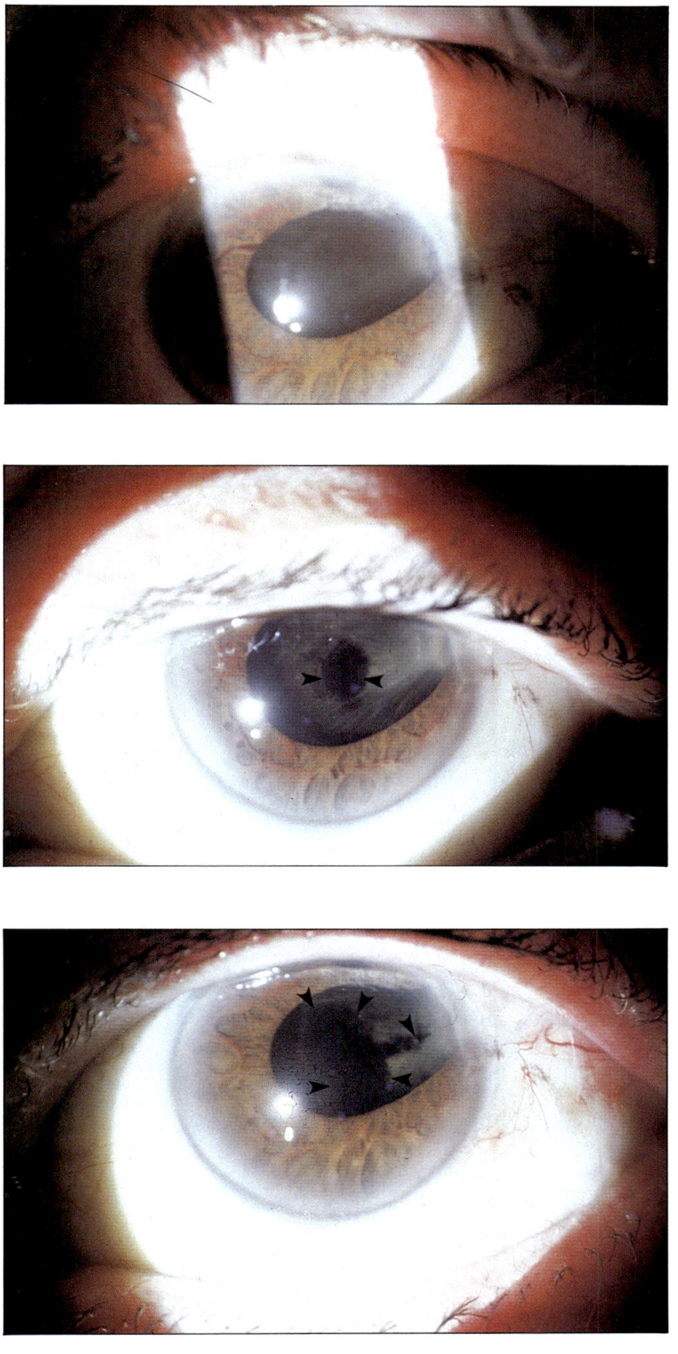

Fig. 39. Aphakic patient post traumatic opacification of the anterior vitreous. **A.** Before laser, traction fibers converge to the corneal wound at 3 o'clock; **B.** after one burst; **C.** after 5 more laser shots from left to right.

Fig. 40. Aphakic patient, traction band going from macular area and iris border at 6 to corneal wound. CME present from 6 weeks, no improvement after steroid therapy. **A.** Before laser treatment, vision 20/200. **B.** After laser section, vision improved within 4 weeks, and stabilized at 20/50. CME looked improved at fluorescein angiography.

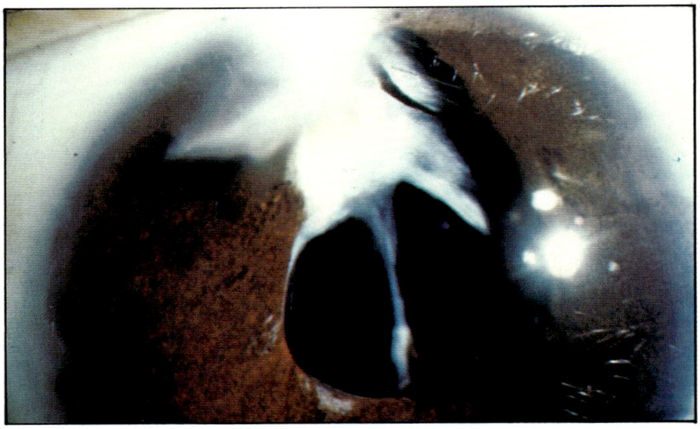

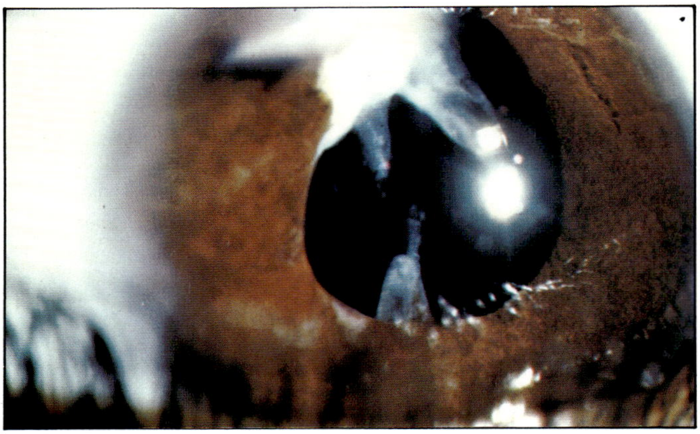

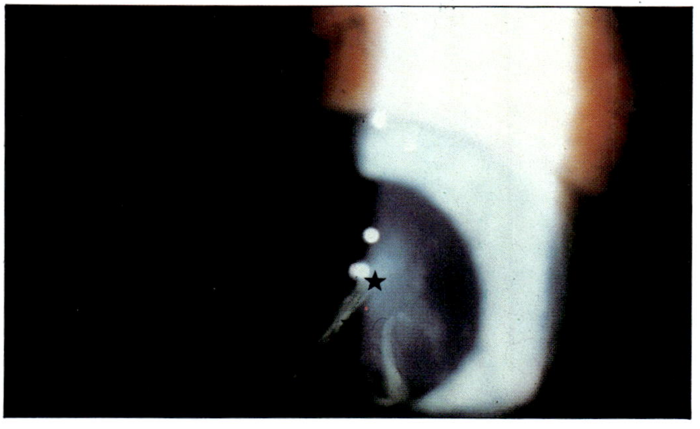

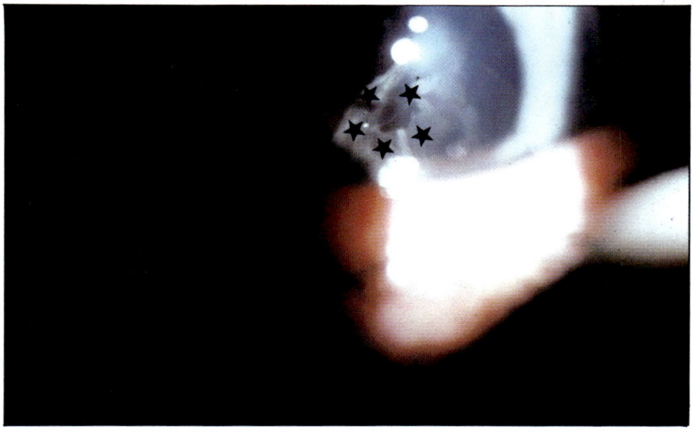

Fig. 41. Retinal detachment and vitreous traction membrane. **A.** Before laser application. **B.** After the third laser burst.

Fig. 42. Retinal detachment, section of traction, phakic patient. **A.** Fixed retinal detachment with strong vitreous tractions. Before pico YAG laser treatment. **B.** During the first session, each band was very tense and was ruptured with a single shot; note plasma bubbles. No laser-induced retinal hemorrhages. **C.** Same day, after the last band has been released. The detached retina is now free and visible in the superior temporal region (arrows); no vitrectomy was necessary at surgery.

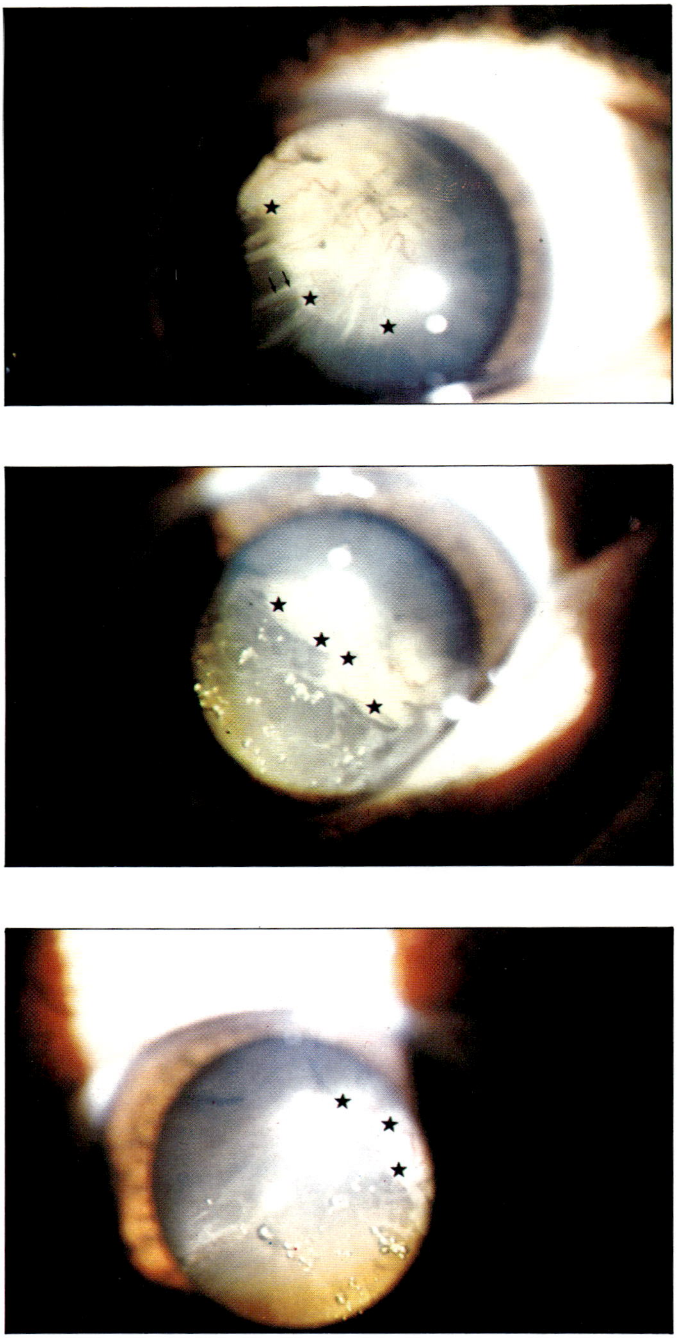

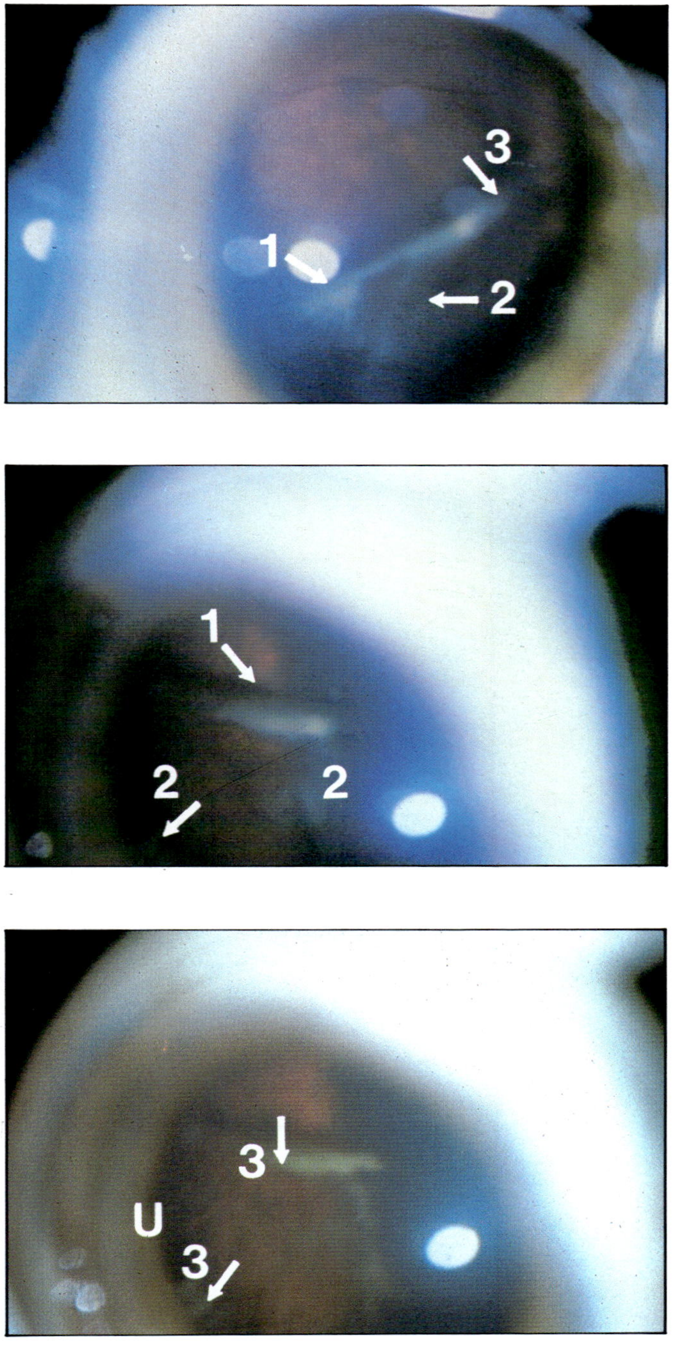

Fig. 43. Section of deep vitreous traction bands. Phakic patient. **A.** Previous to laser section. Retina-to-retina traction band. Main branch oriented from 10 to 4 o'clock. Situation 1 millimeter (3 diopters) from the retina. 1-2-3 indicates the site of laser section to be done. Note normal retinal vessels at the superior part. **B.** Section 1 necessitates 5 laser bursts. Section 2 was obtained after 2 shots. Releasing branches 2 and 1 result in liberation of the band which, now free, is located in 2 upper position, so hiding the retinal vessels. **C.** After section in 3 the traction band has become independent from the retina and floats more anteriorly in the vitreous. No hemorrhages, no retinal swelling, no modifications at fluorescein angiography were laser-induced.

Fig. 44A. Congenital Cataract. Opacified capsule 15 years after surgery. Before laser treatment vision reduced to light perception.

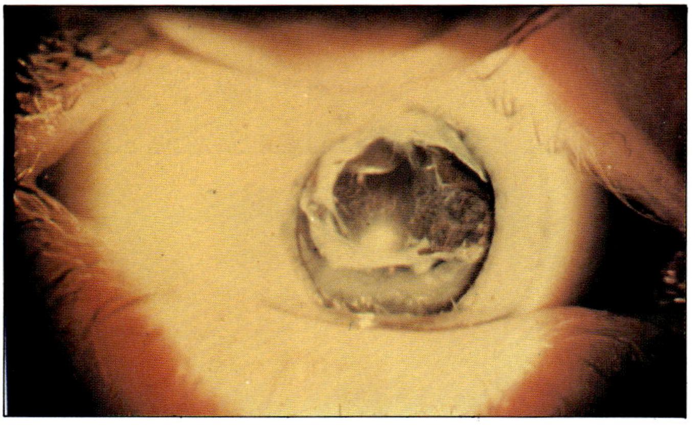

Fig. 44B. Congenital Cataract. After 3 laser shots and 2 days after laser session, vision 20/20 with aphakic glasses.

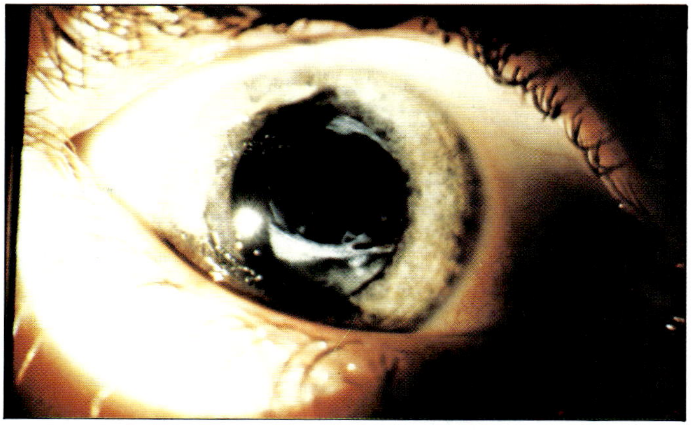

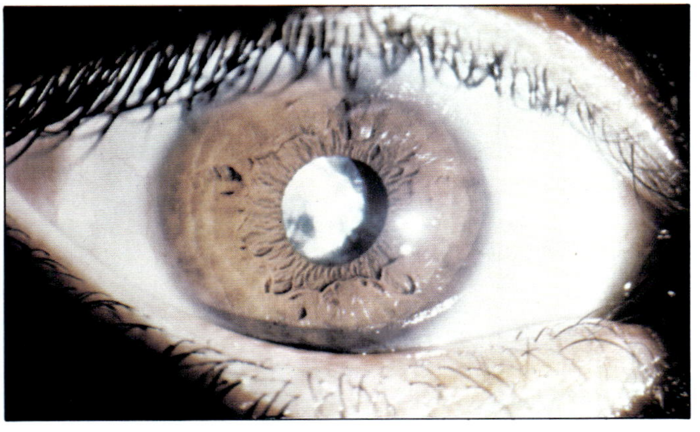

Fig. 45A. Contusive cataract in a 4-year-old child (seen 2 years after traumatism) before laser treatment.

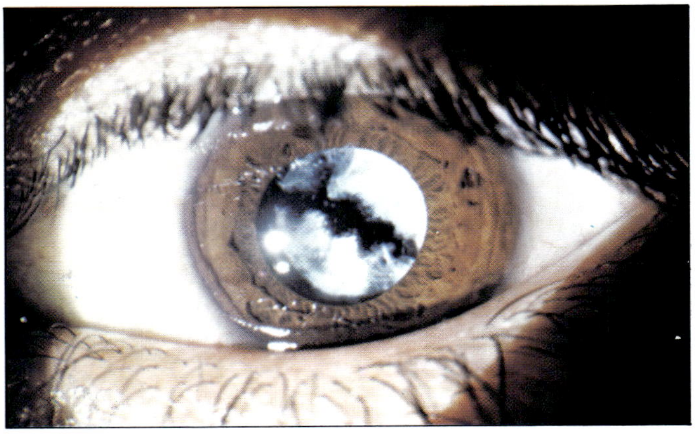

Fig. 45B. Contusive cataract after one session and 62 shots.

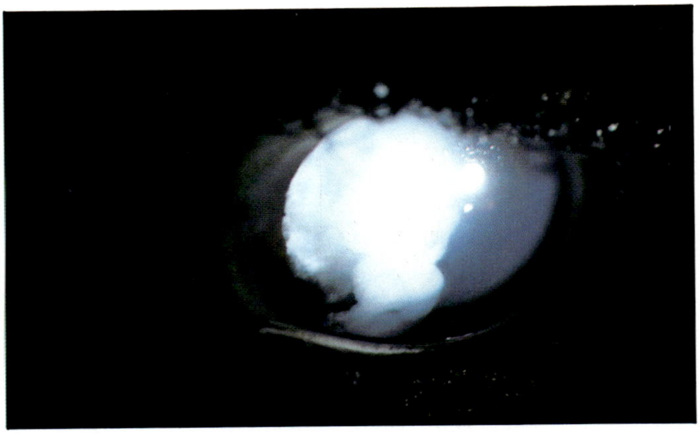

Fig. 46A. Child, 2 years old. Congenital hypermature soft cataract; contraindication to general anesthesia. After five vertical laser shots on the anterior capsule, lens material spreads down in the anterior chamber.

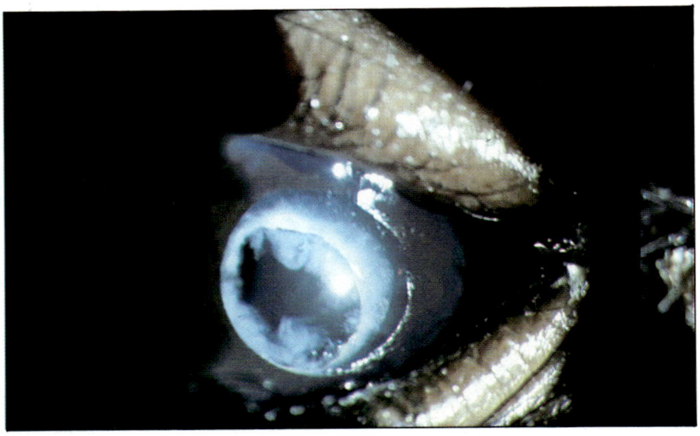

Fig. 46B. Ten days later lens material has cleared up and no inflammatory reaction was present.

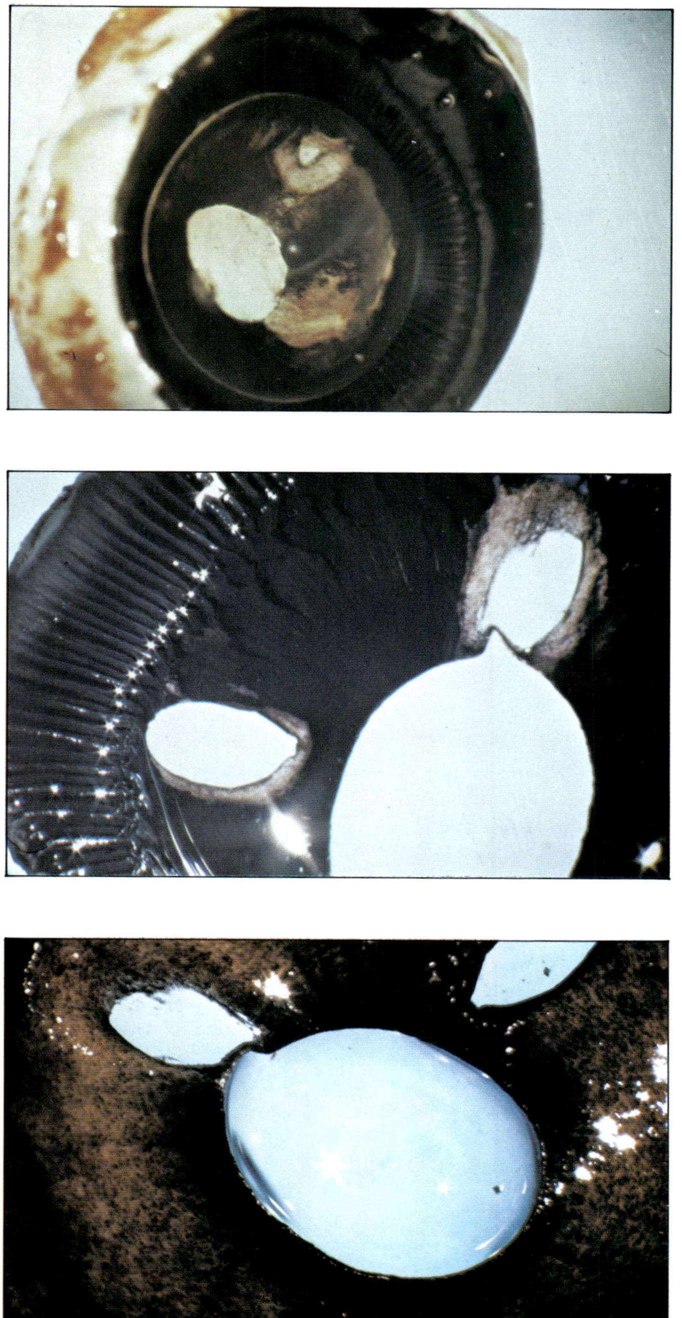

Fig. 47 A–C. YAG nanosecond iridectomy (rabbits' eye).

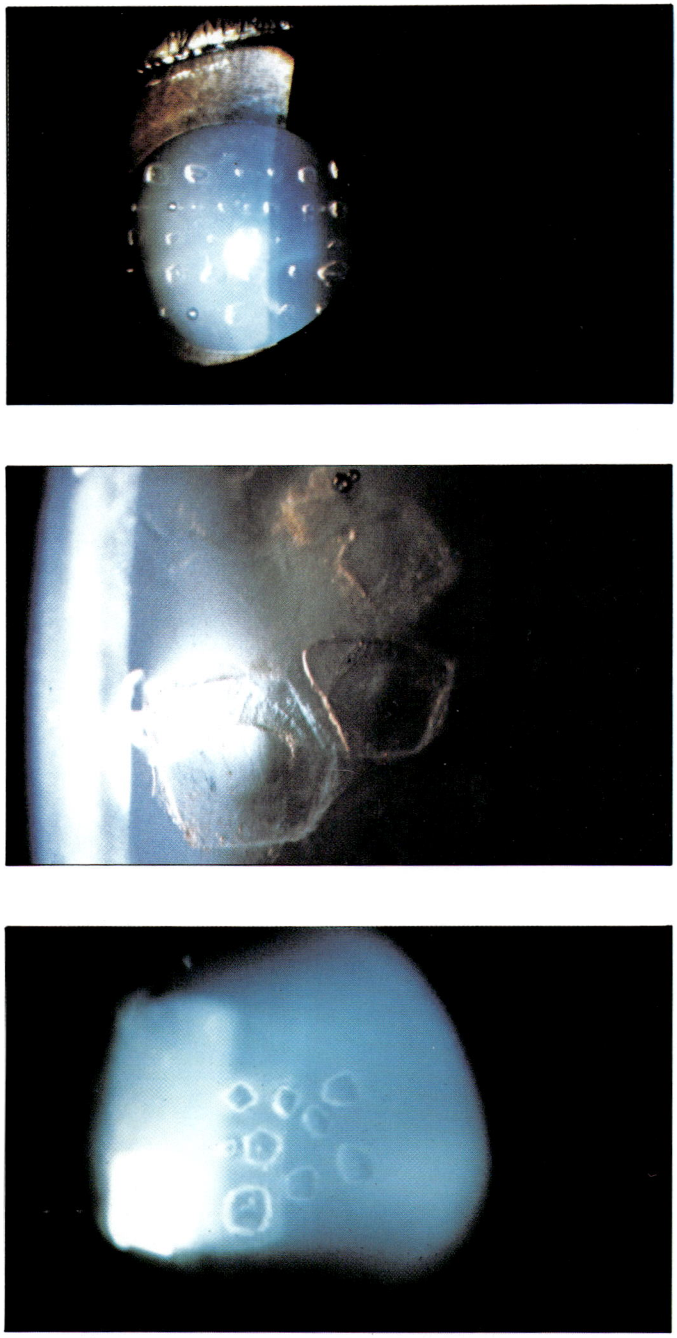

Fig. 48. YAG laser anterior capsulotomy (human). **A.** Picolaser anterior capsulotomy. **B, C.** Nanolaser anterior capsulotomy.

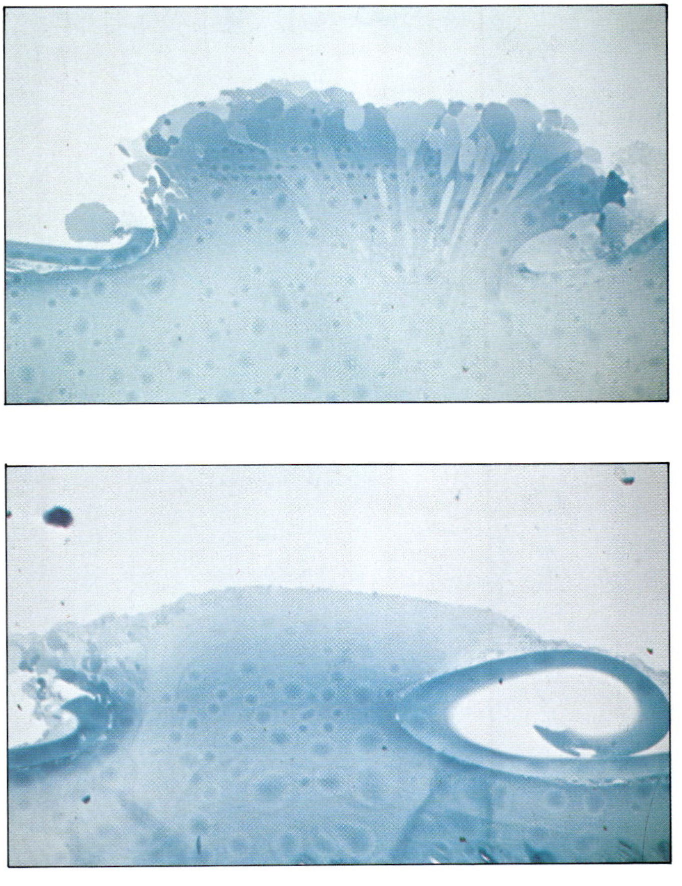

Fig. 49. Pathology of YAG induced capsulotomy . **A.** Picolaser induced capsulotomy. **B.** Nanolaser induced capsulotomy.

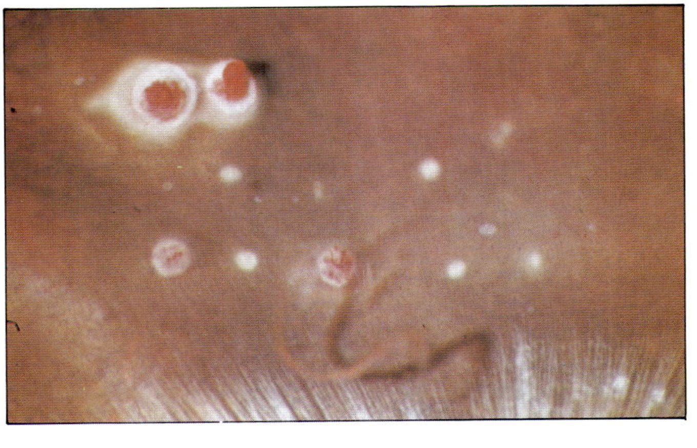

Fig. 50. Nanosecond induced lesions on the rabbit's retina. Shot located at 2mm-3mm from the retina.

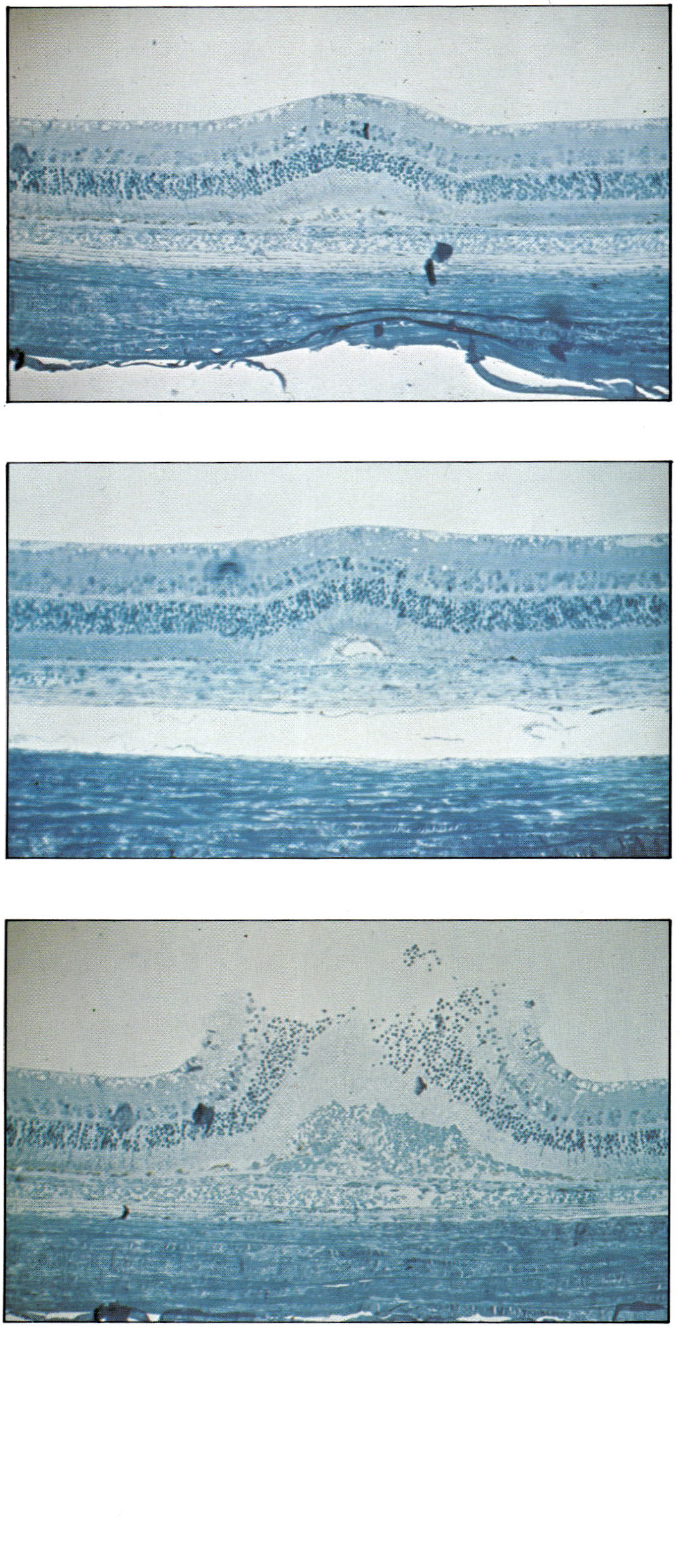

Fig. 51. Nano Q-switched laser-induced retinal lesions. **A.** Shot located at 3 mm from the retina; power 1.5 mjoules; Optical breakdown present. **B.** Monomode modification shot located at 2 mm from retina; power 3 to 3.5 mjoules; optical breakdown present. **C.** Multimode modification of the Q-switched nanosecond. Shot located at 3 mm from the retina; power 3 to 3.5 millijoules.

Side Effects

Laser	Iridectomy	Capsulotomy
Q-switch	no corneal side effects with contact-lens defect of pigment-epithelium enlargement of primary effect opacification of anterior-lens capsule (focal)	no retinal side effects no corneal side effects with contact-lens corneal side effects without contact-lens
mode-locked	iridectomies are not possible	no retinal side effects no corneal side effects without contact-lens

Fig. 52. Compared side-effects of Q-switched nanolasers and modelocked monomode picosecond lasers.

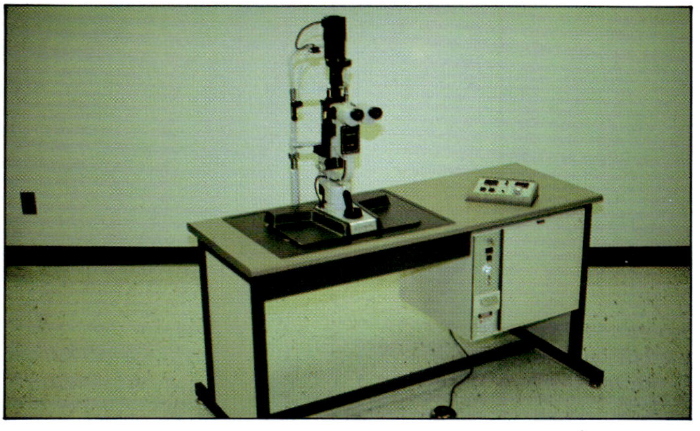

Fig. 53. AMO Q-switched YAG laser.

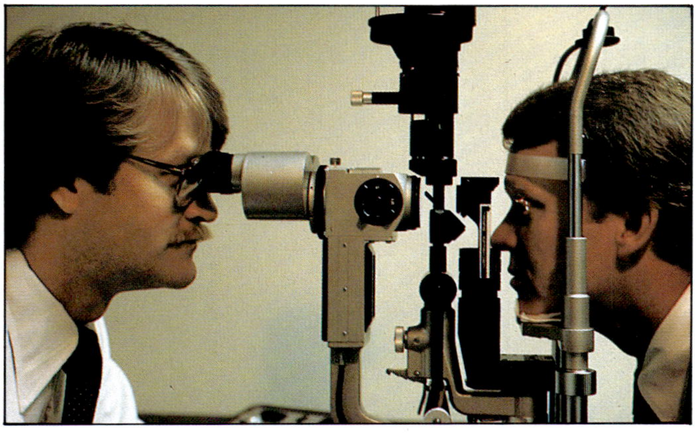

Fig 54. Patient in position at laser.

Fig. 55. First aphakic patient with a secondary membrane, pre-YAG.

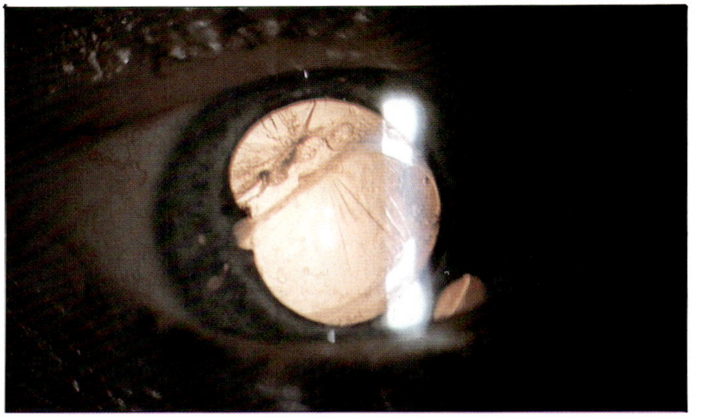

Fig. 56. First aphakic secondary membrane, post-YAG.

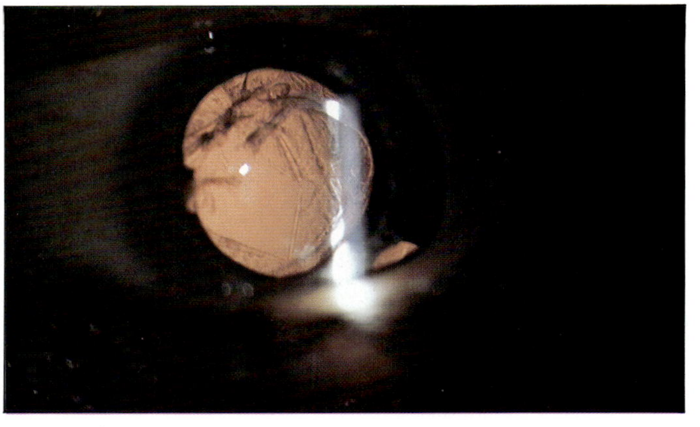

Fig. 57. Second aphakic patient with a secondary membrane, pre-YAG.

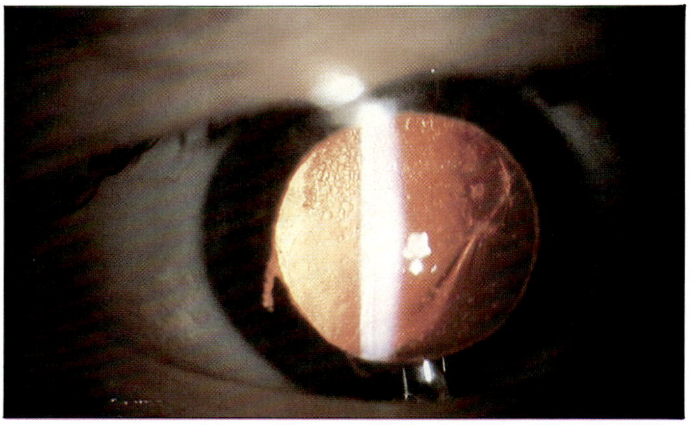

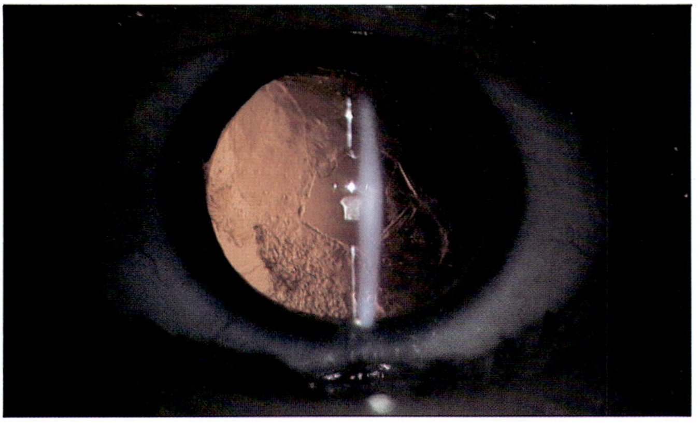

Fig. 58. Second aphakic patient with a secondary membrane, post-YAG.

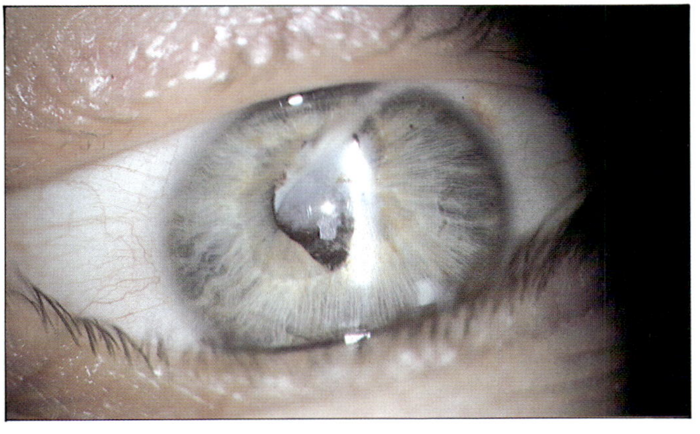

Fig. 59. Aphakic patient, very dense secondary membrane, pre-YAG.

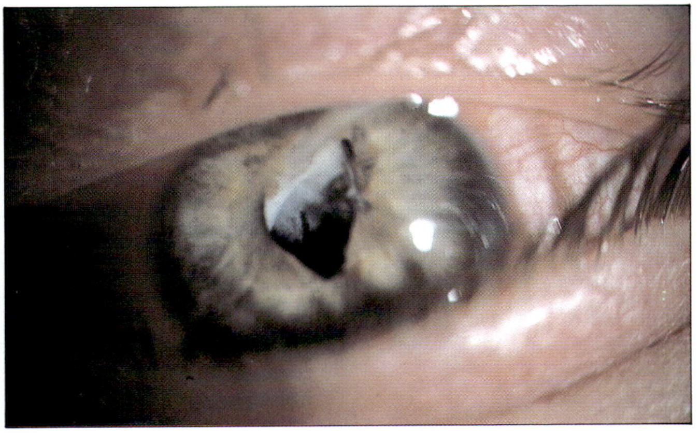

Fig. 60. Aphakic patient, very dense secondary membrane, post-YAG.

Fig. 61 Pseudophakos with a Kratz IOL secondary membrane, pre-YAG.

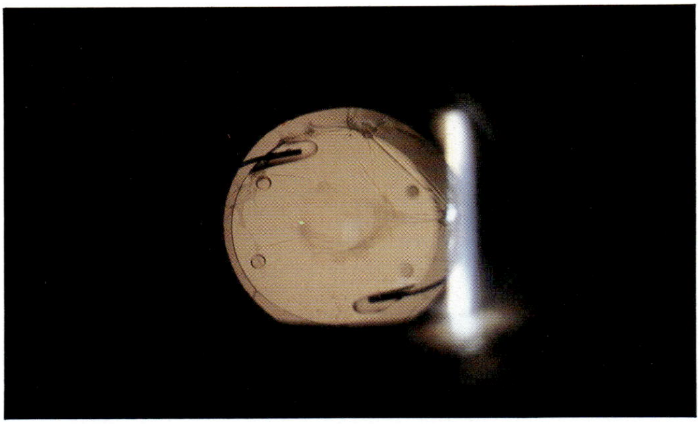

Fig. 62. Pseudophakos with a Kratz IOL secondary membrane, post-YAG.

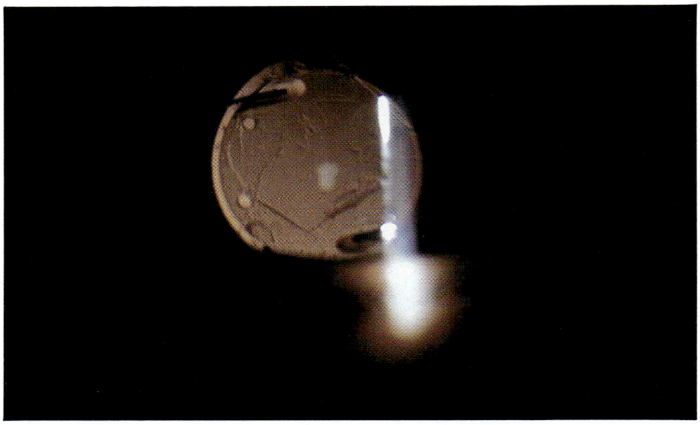

Fig. 63. Pseudophakos dense secondary membrane, pre-YAG.

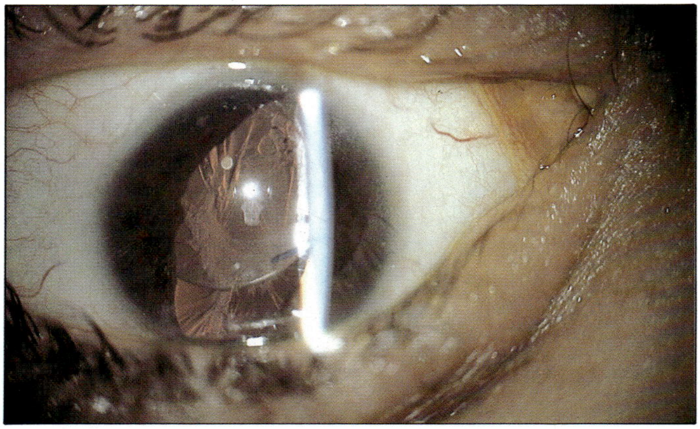

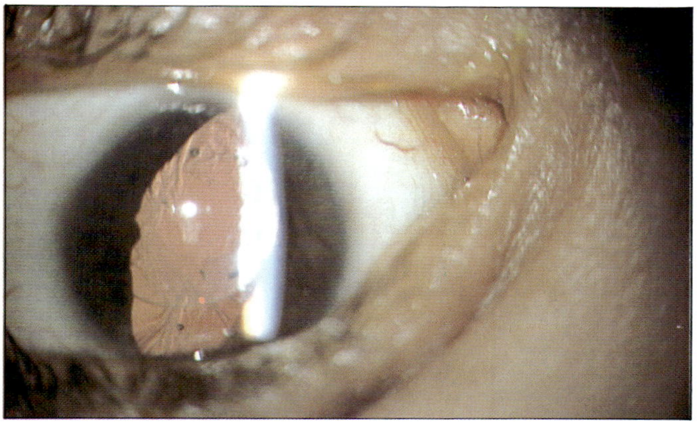

Fig. 64. Pseudophakos dense secondary membrane, post-YAG.

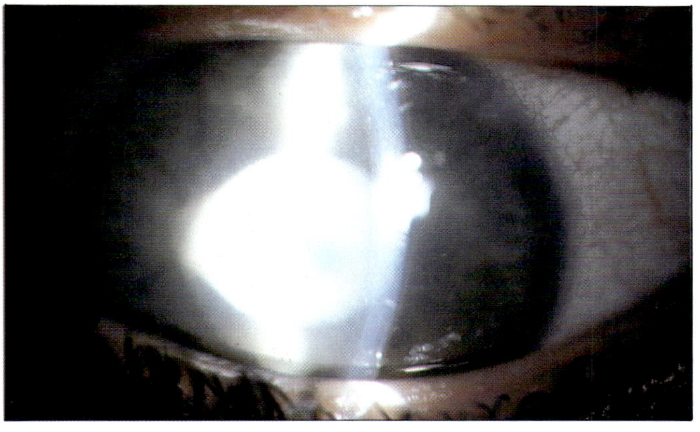

Fig. 65. Glaucoma patient showing marked inflammation post capsulotomy with residual cortex, post-YAG.

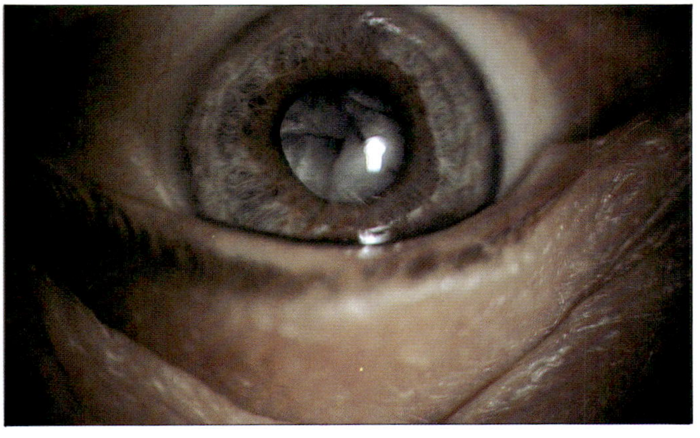

Fig. 66. Pre-YAG aphakic cortical material.

Fig. 67. Post-YAG aphakic cortical material.

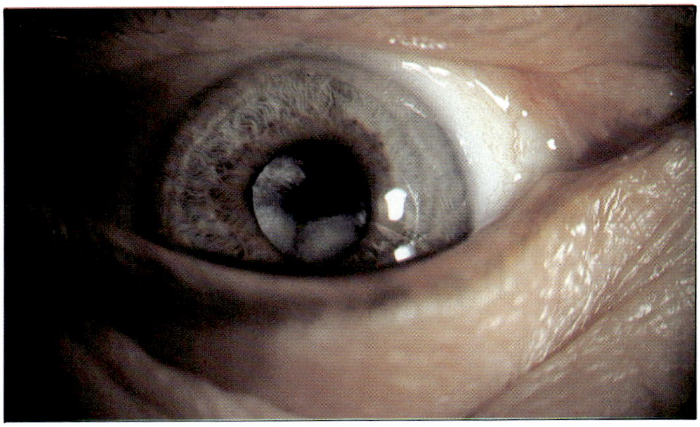

Fig. 68. Lysis of membrane to cornea, pre-YAG.

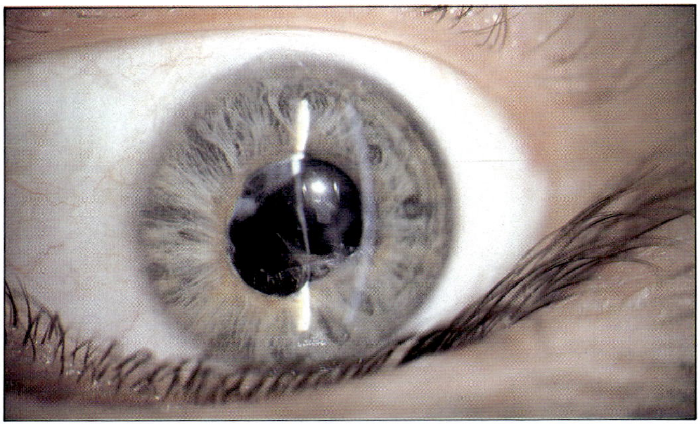

Fig. 69. Lysis of membrane to cornea, post YAG.

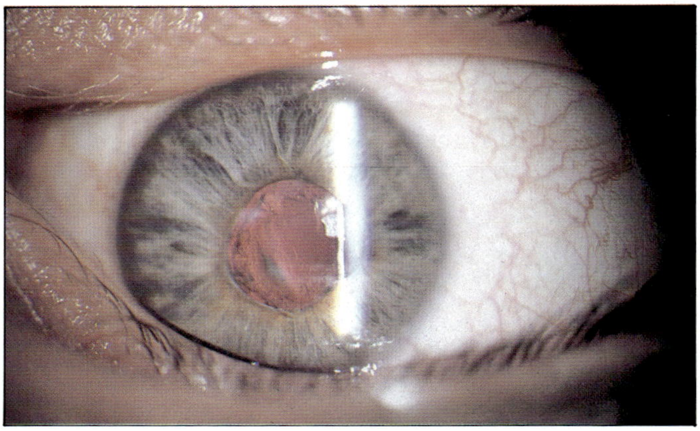

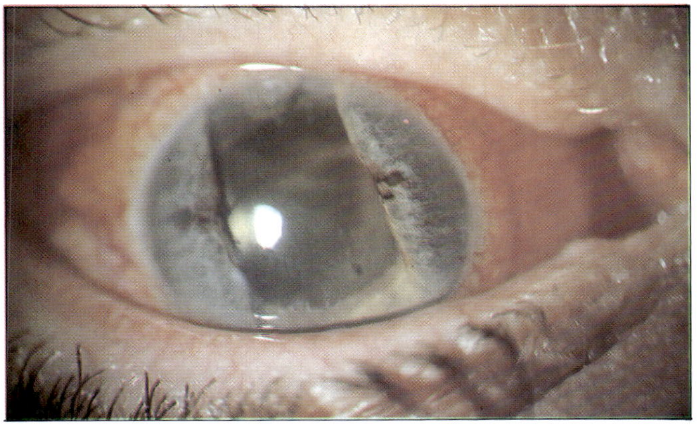

Fig. 70. Patient with pupillary block where iridectomies were made with the YAG laser.

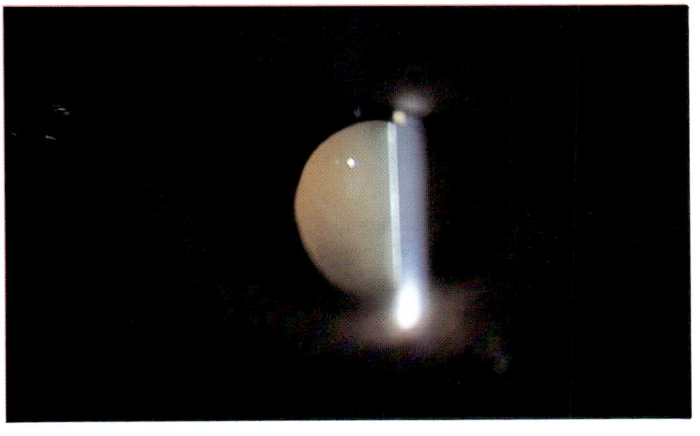

Fig. 71. Pre-YAG vitreous haze.

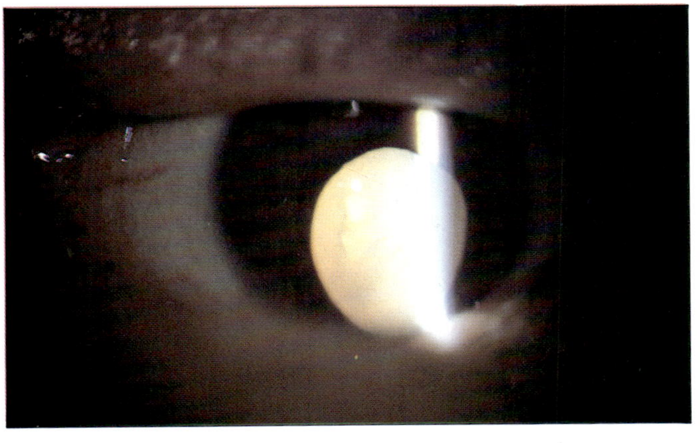

Fig. 72. Post-YAG vitreous haze.

ATLAS OF PATHOLOGY

ATLAS Figs. A–D. Possible beam distortions according to the position.

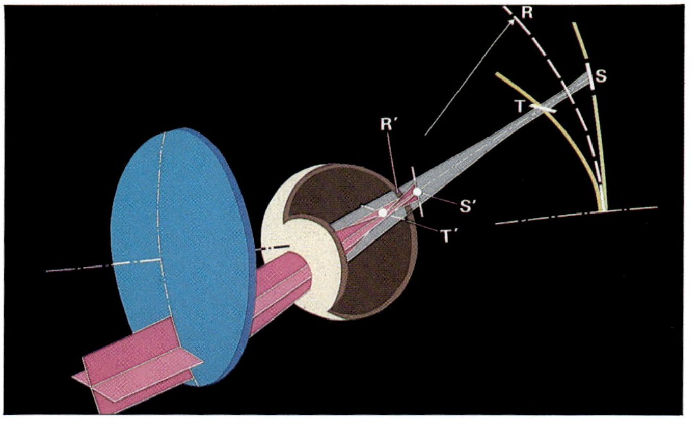

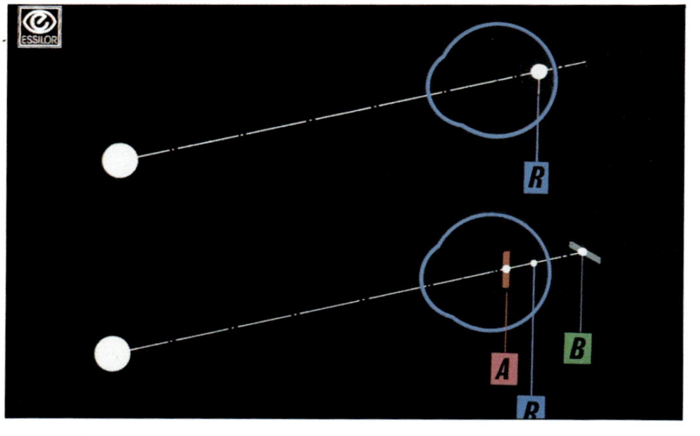

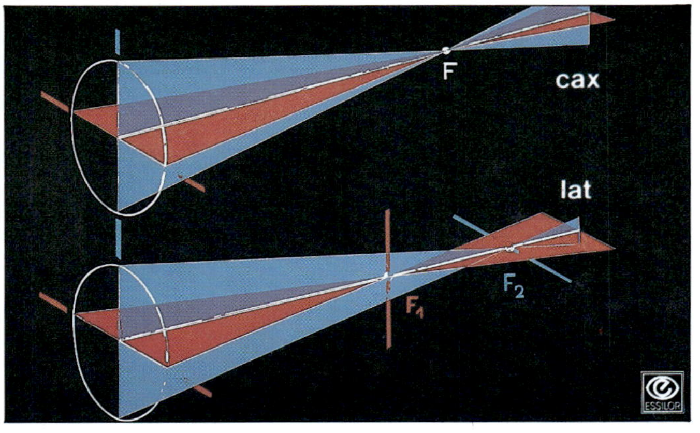
F
cax
lat
F1
F2
ESSILOR

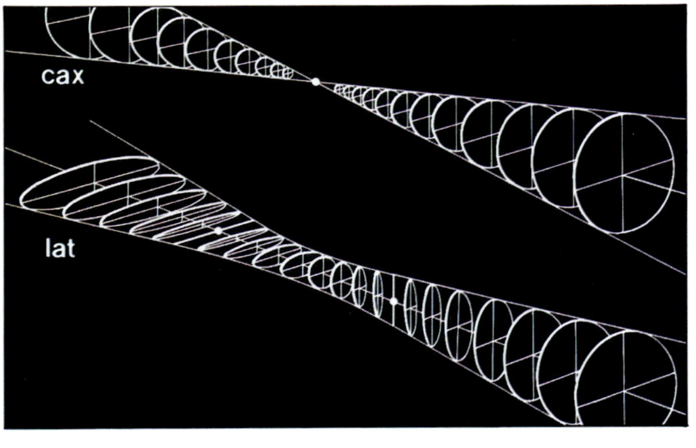
cax
lat

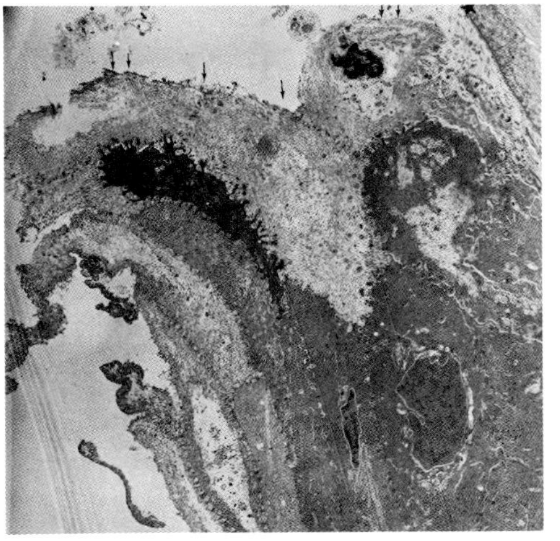

ATLAS Fig. E. Pico laser induced corneal lesion; coaxial shot on the corneal epithelium. Corneal epithelium at the site of the shot (transmission em). Magnification 2550: one micron = 2.55 cm. Clear section, epithelium vaporized (arrow). The basal membrane is normal. Picnosis of the nuclei. Slight epithelial detachment. Nuclei become normal at the third cell.

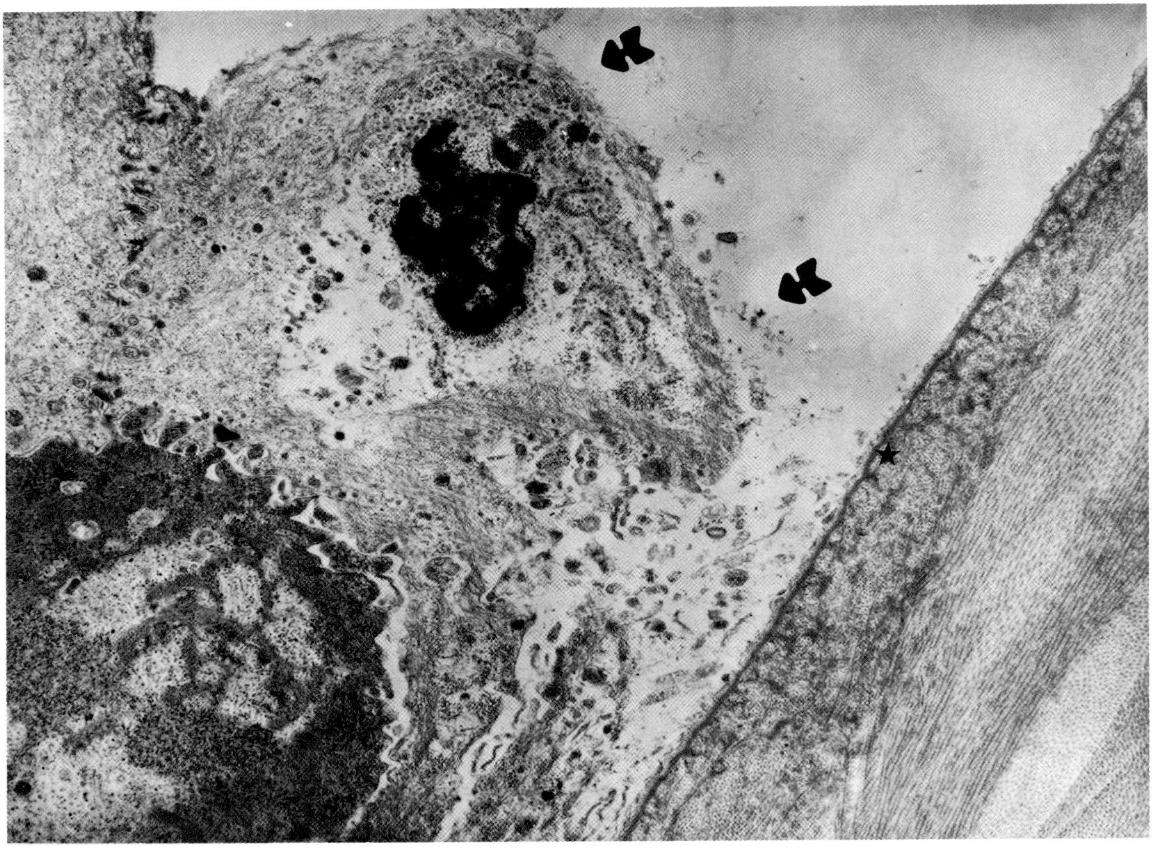

ATLAS Fig. F. Pico laser induced corneal lesion; coaxial shot on the corneal epithelium (transmission em). Magnification 12,000: one micron = 12 cm. The basal membrane is normal. Lesion well limited; arrow. The neighboring cell's nucleus is in picnosis; the next cell's nucleus is slightly modified. There are modifications of the cell's limiting membranes, no further than the second cell from the lesion. The stroma is swollen and the underlying Bowman's membrane is normal.

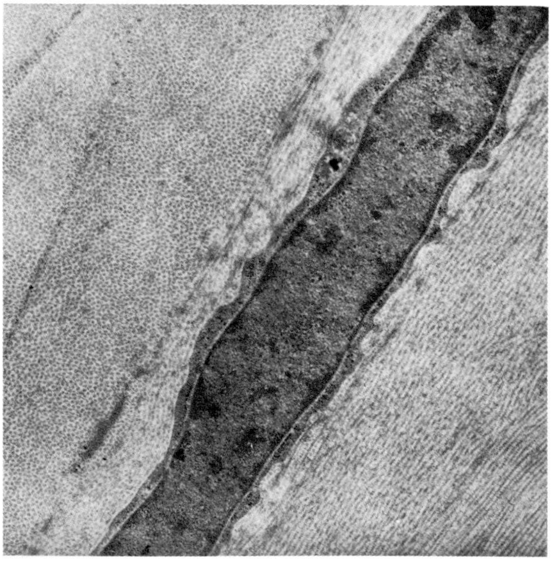

ATLAS Fig. G. Pico laser induced corneal lesion; coaxial shot on the epithelium at 83 microns from the center of the burst (transmission em). Magnification $\times$ 24,000. One micron = 24 cm. At 83 microns from the center of the focal destruction, a normal keratocyte and normal stroma.

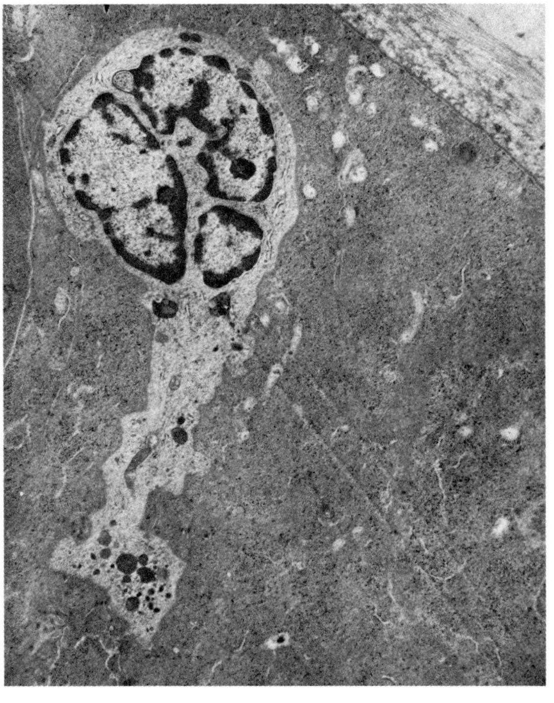

ATLAS Fig. H. Pico laser induced corneal lesion; coaxial shot on the corneal epithelium. At 166 microns from the burst (transmission em). Magnification $\times$ 12,000. One micron = 12 cm. At 166 microns away from the laser shot; Normal axon in normal stroma.

ATLAS Fig. I. Pico laser induced corneal lesion; coaxial shot on the corneal epithelium. At the site of the lesion (transmission em). Magnification 24,000. One micron = 24 cm. At the site of the lesion; normal stroma under a destroyed basal membrane.

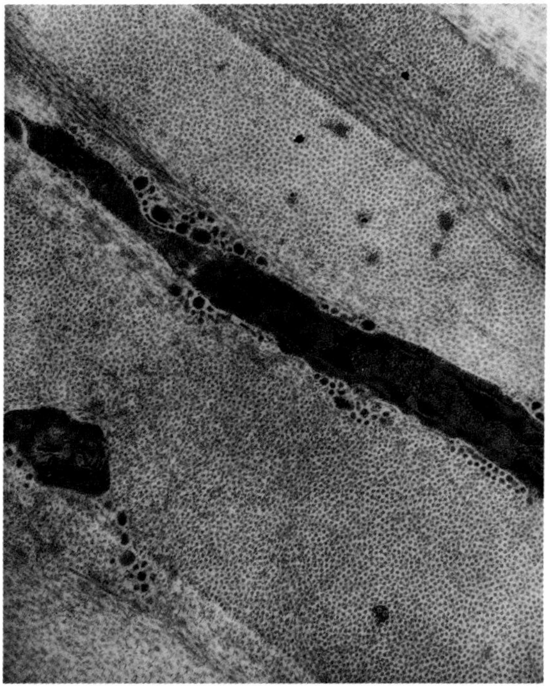

ATLAS Fig. J. Pico laser induced corneal lesion; coaxial shot on the corneal endothelium (transmission em). Magnification 14,000. One micron = 14 cm. Endothelium opposite to the epithelial shot. The endothelium is normal.

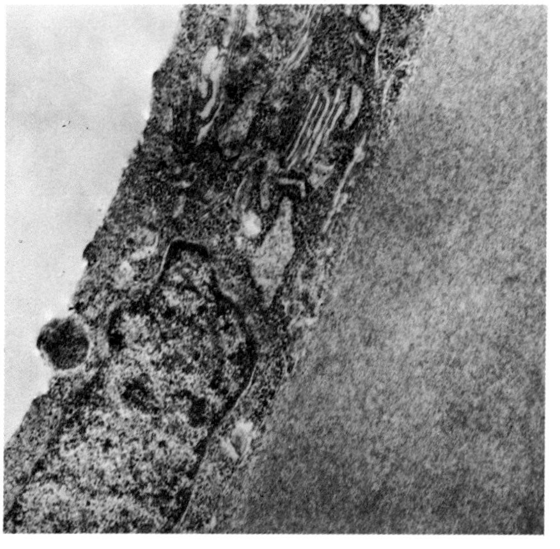

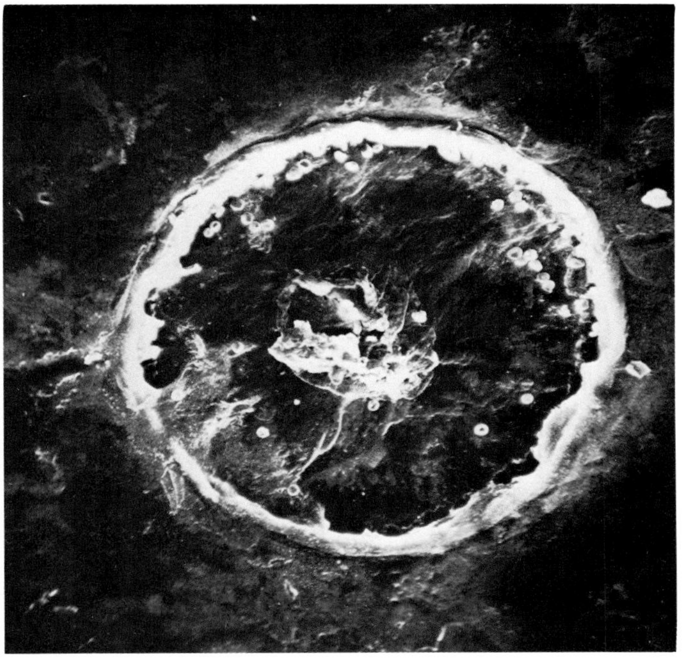

ATLAS Fig. K. Scanning electron microscopy study of modelocked ND YAG laser shots on the rabbit cornea. Direct shot on the corneal epithelium—MAG × 300 1 cm = 35 microns. a—size of the lesion: the lesion is perfectly circular and limited to 230 to 260 microns width. The center of the lesion (site of the optical breakdown) is 70 to 80 microns wide. When the shot is coaxial the lesion is a perfect circle; the more oblique the laser beam the more elipsoïd the destruction. b—thickness: the surface of the lesion is flat; the underlying stroma is normal; the corneal endothelium is destroyed.

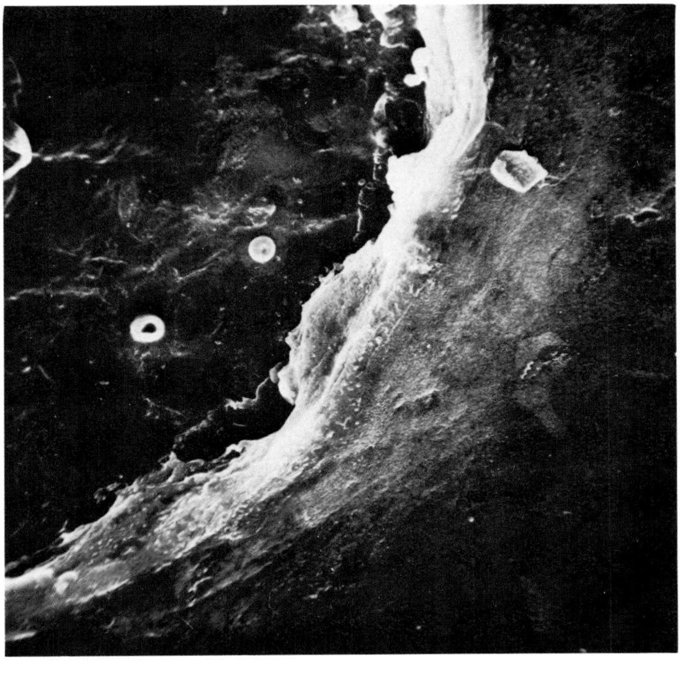

ATLAS Fig. L. Scanning electron microscopy study of modelocked ND YAG laser shots on the rabbit cornea. Direct shot on the corneal endothelium —MAG × 800 1 cm = 13 microns. Direct shot on corneal epithelium: borders of the lesion. c—The limits of the shot: the limits of the shot are perfectly well outlined, even when the laser beam is not coaxial. The lesion is surrounded by a ring (1 or 2 cells large), of slightly swollen cells. The surrounding corneal epithelium is totally normal.

ATLAS Fig. M. Scanning electron microscopy study of modelocked ND YAG laser shots on the rabbit cornea. Direct shot on corneal epithelium central area MAG × 800 1 cm = 13 microns. d—The central area: the central area corresponds to the shot zone itself and is grossly circular. It is composed of a shrunken stromal tissue forming a central mound.

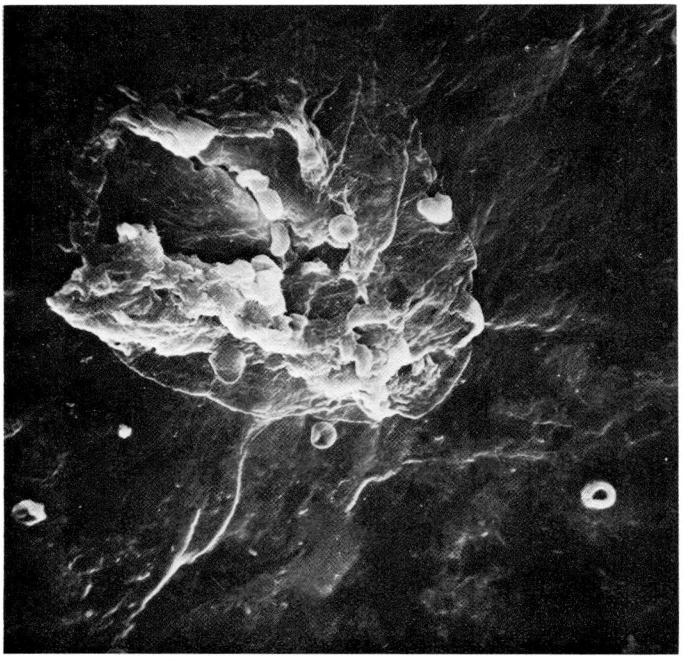

ATLAS Fig. N. Scanning electron microscopy study of modelocked ND YAG laser shots on the rabbit cornea. Direct shot on the corneal epithelium. MAG × 3,000. 1 cm = 3.5 microns. Central zone; tissue totally shrunken.

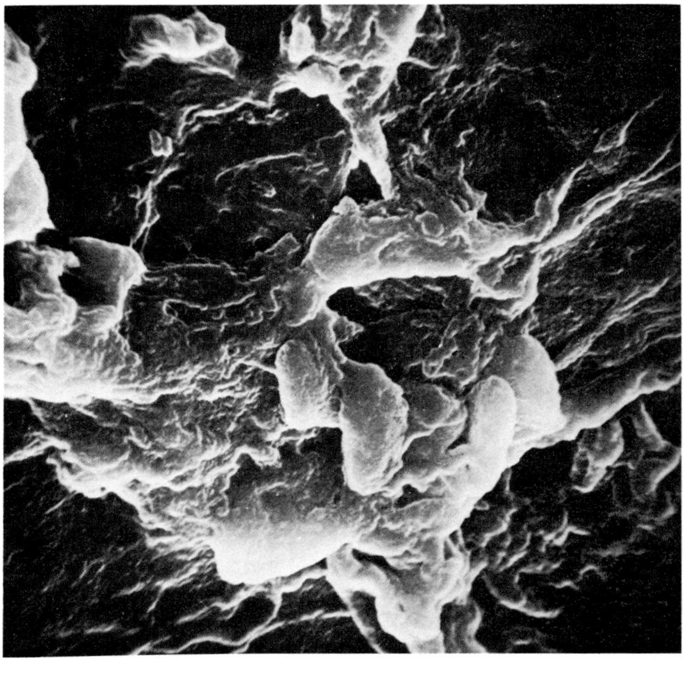

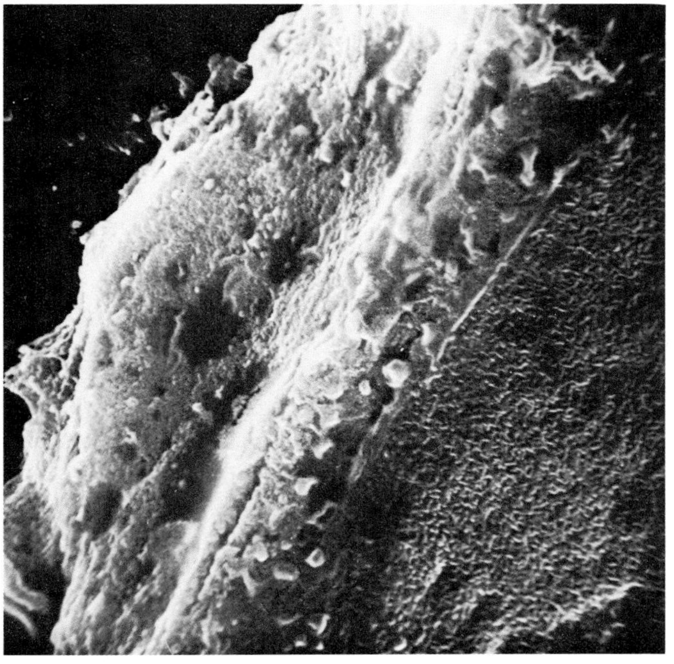

ATLAS Fig. O. Scanning electron microscopy study of the modelocked ND YAG laser shots on the rabbit cornea. Direct shot on the corneal epithelium. MAG × 3,000. 1 cm = 3.5 microns. Peripheral zone with diffusion of the shock wave pushing the endothelium into a ring of 4 times the diameter of the impact zone.

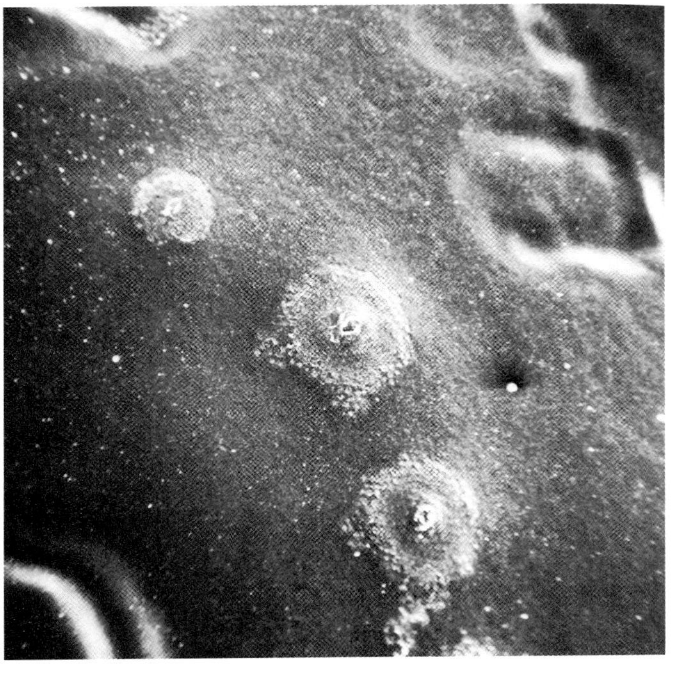

ATLAS Fig. P. Scanning electron microscopy study of the modelocked ND YAG picolaser shots on the rabbit cornea. Direct shot on the cornea endothelium. a: Shot in coaxial position. × 70: shrinkage of the central part. 1 cm = 140 microns.

ATLAS Fig. Q. Scanning electron microscopy study of the modelocked ND YAG picolaser shots on the rabbit cornea. Direct shot on the cornea endothelium. a: Shot in coaxial position. × 200: Perfectly level limited round lesion. 1 cm = 40 microns.

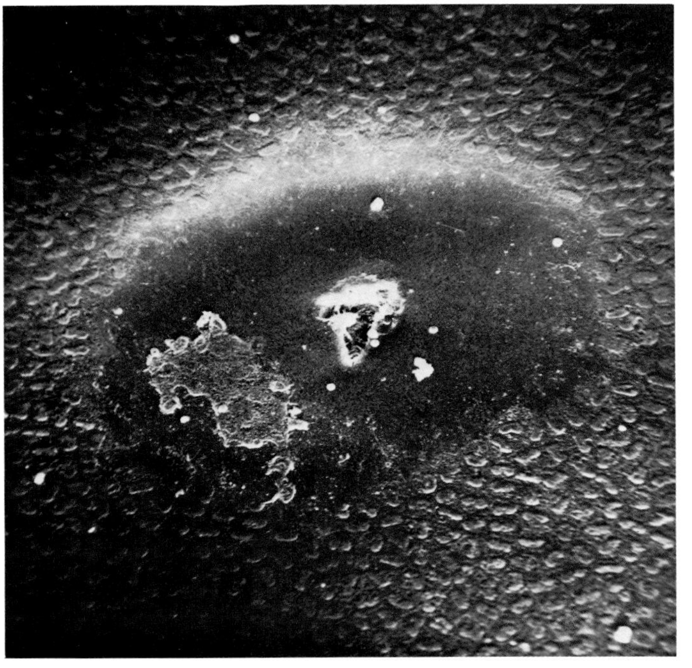

ATLAS Fig. R. Scanning electron microscopy study of the modelocked ND YAG picolaser shots on the rabbit cornea. Direct shot on the cornea endothelium. a: Shot in coaxial position. × 3000: no transition zone between normal and destroyed tissue. Typical monomode modelocked laser-induced lesion on the endothelium. 1 cm = 13 microns.

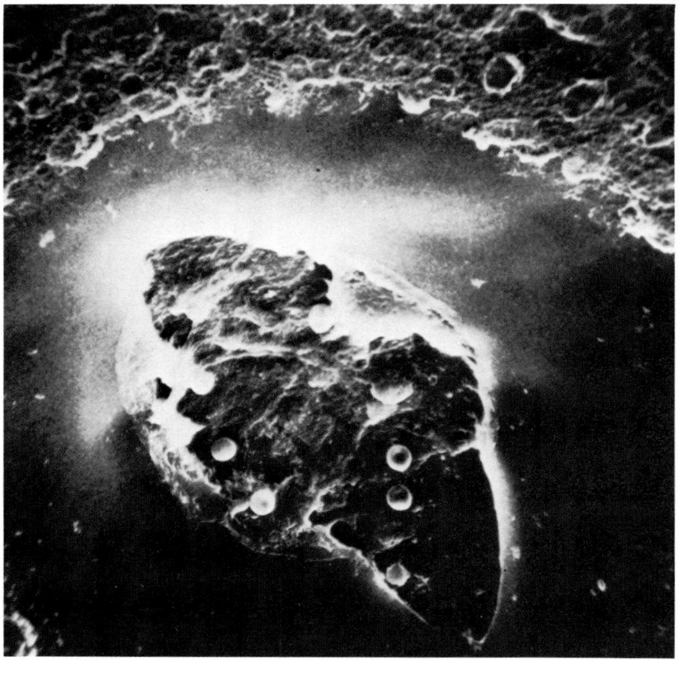

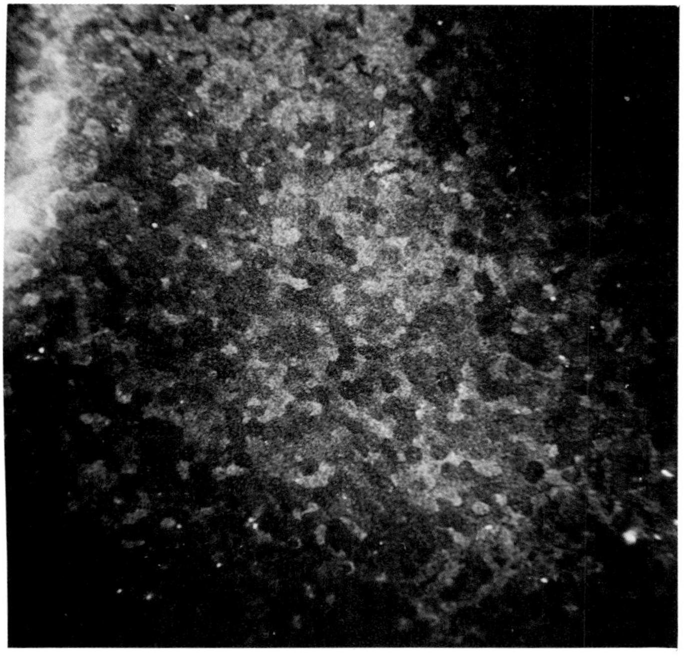

ATLAS Fig. S. Scanning electron microscopy study of the modelocked ND YAG picolaser shots on the rabbit cornea. Direct shot on the cornea endothelium. a: Shot in coaxial position. $\times$ 70: corneal epithelium in the axis of the endothelial burst is normal. 1 cm = 140 microns.

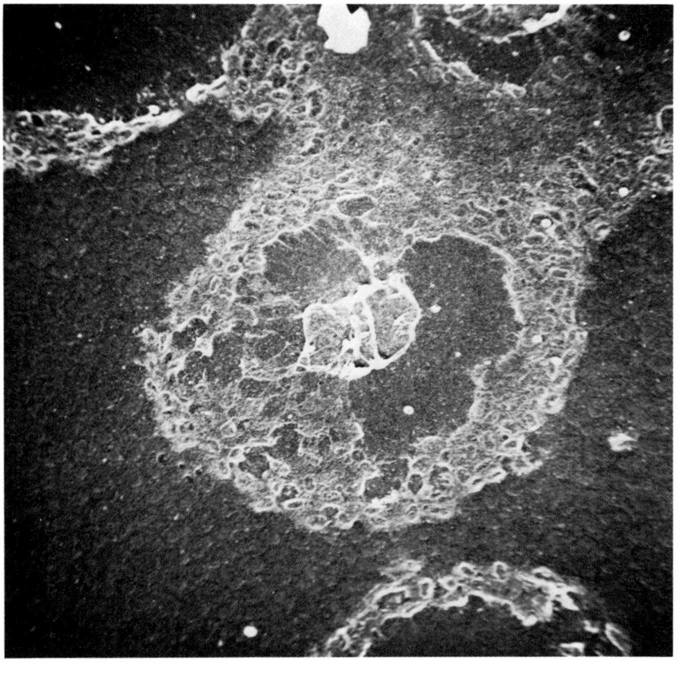

ATLAS Fig. T. Scanning electron microscopy study of the modelocked ND YAG picolaser shots on the rabbit cornea. Direct shot on the cornea endothelium. b: Shot in lateral position. $\times$ 200: the shrunken central zone has become oval: a larger ring of swollen cells surrounds the destroyed tissue. The general shape of the destruction is more ovalized. 1 cm = 40 microns.

ATLAS Fig. U. Scanning electron microscopy study of the modelocked ND YAG picolaser shots on the rabbit cornea. Direct shot on the cornea endothelium. b: Shot in lateral position. × 200: corneal epithelium opposite to the endothelial burst is the site of a superficial oval lesion. 1 cm = 40 microns.

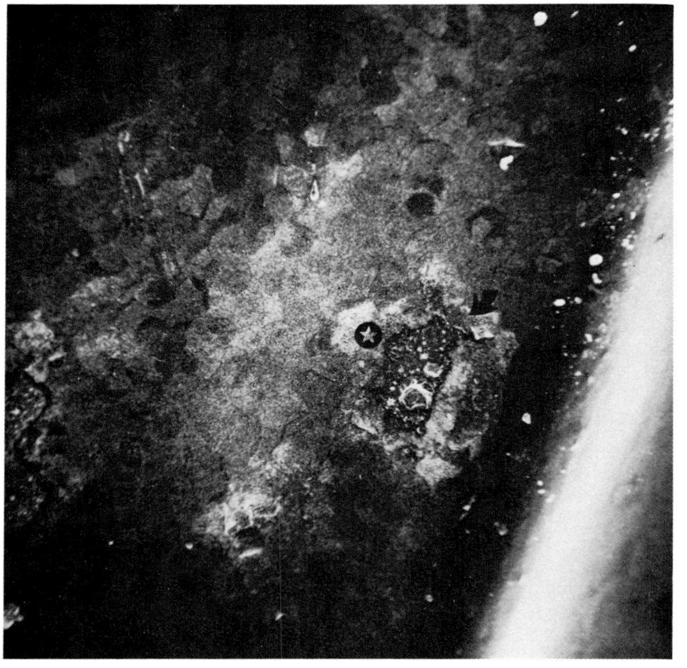

ATLAS Fig. V. Scanning electron microscopy study of the modelocked ND YAG picolaser shots on the rabbit cornea. Direct shot on the cornea endothelium. b: Shot in lateral position. × 300: both endothelium-epithelium demonstrate an ovalized zone of destruction. 1 cm = 35 microns.

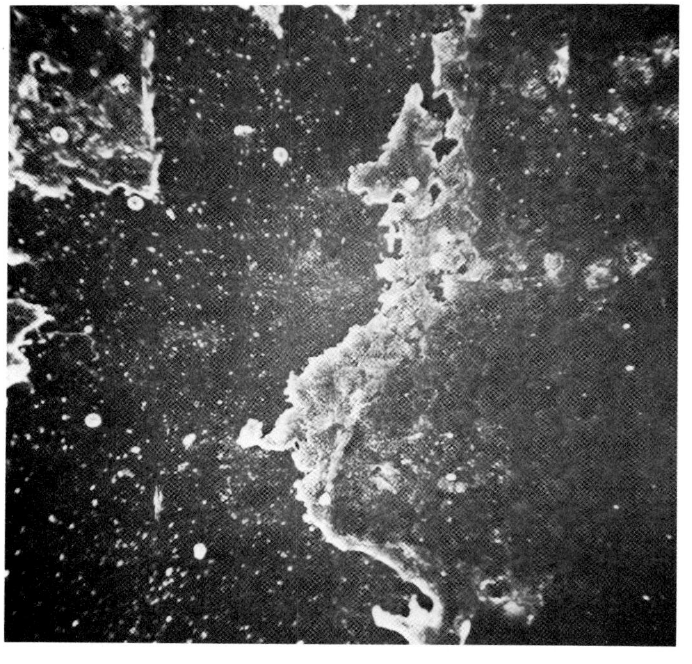

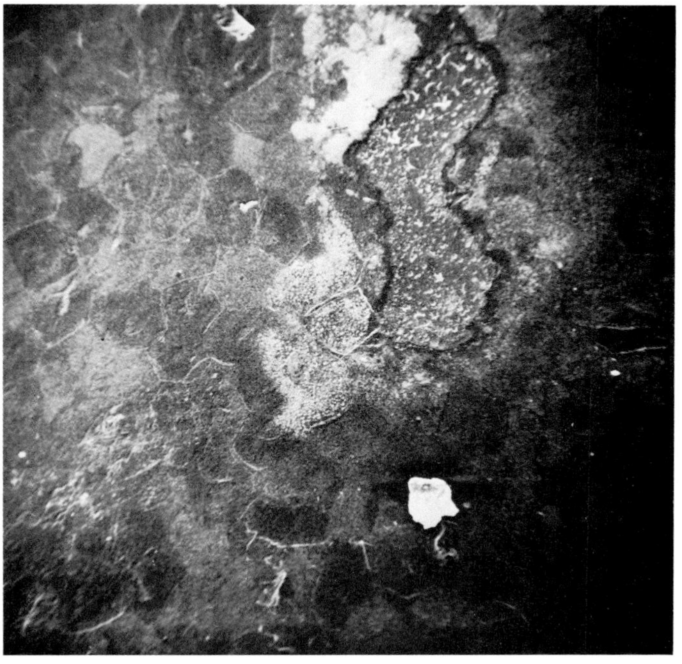

ATLAS Fig. W. Scanning electron microscopy study of the modelocked ND YAG picolaser shots on the rabbit cornea. Direct shot on the cornea endothelium. b: Shot in lateral position. The epithelial lesions appear to be less extensive than the endothelial destruction.

ATLAS Fig. X. Picolaser monomode modelocked induced lesion on the endothelium: coaxial shot. Anterior diffusion of the shock wave. Transmission microscopy. At the site of the burst; endothelium has broken. Stroma in the vicinity is swollen.

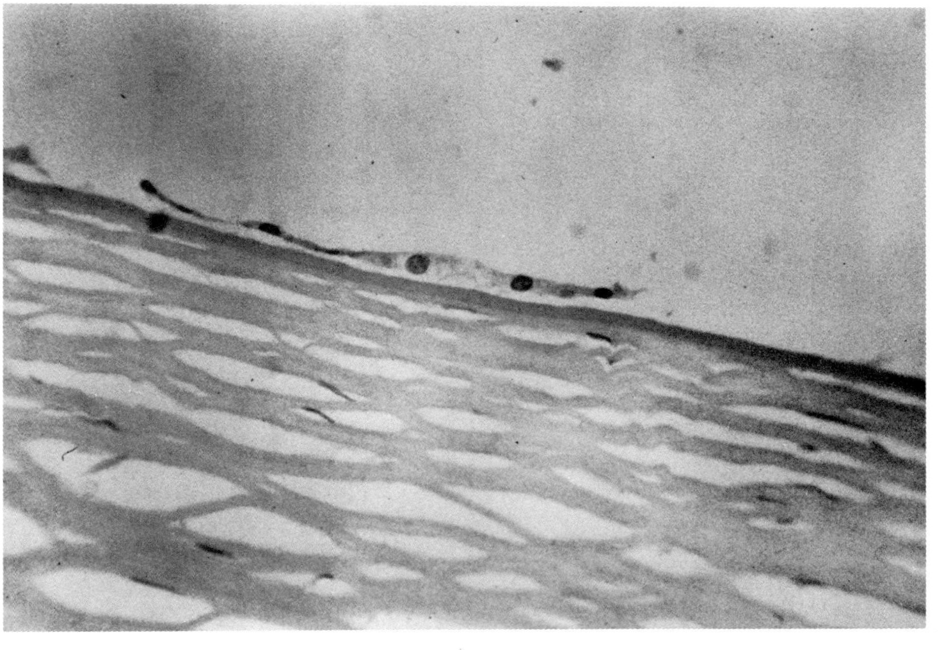

ATLAS Fig. Y. Scanning electron microscope study of modelocked neodymium YAG laser shots on the rabbit lens. Study of the trajectory of a coaxial shot into the rabbit lens cortex: external view. 16 × magnification. The lesion is a well-circumscribed round hole of approximately 90 microns in diameter.

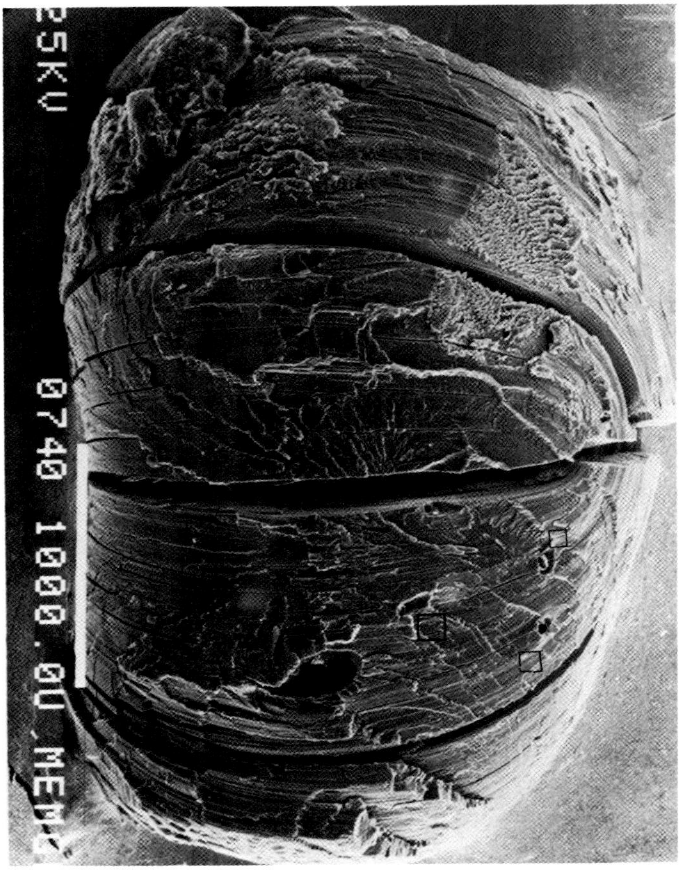

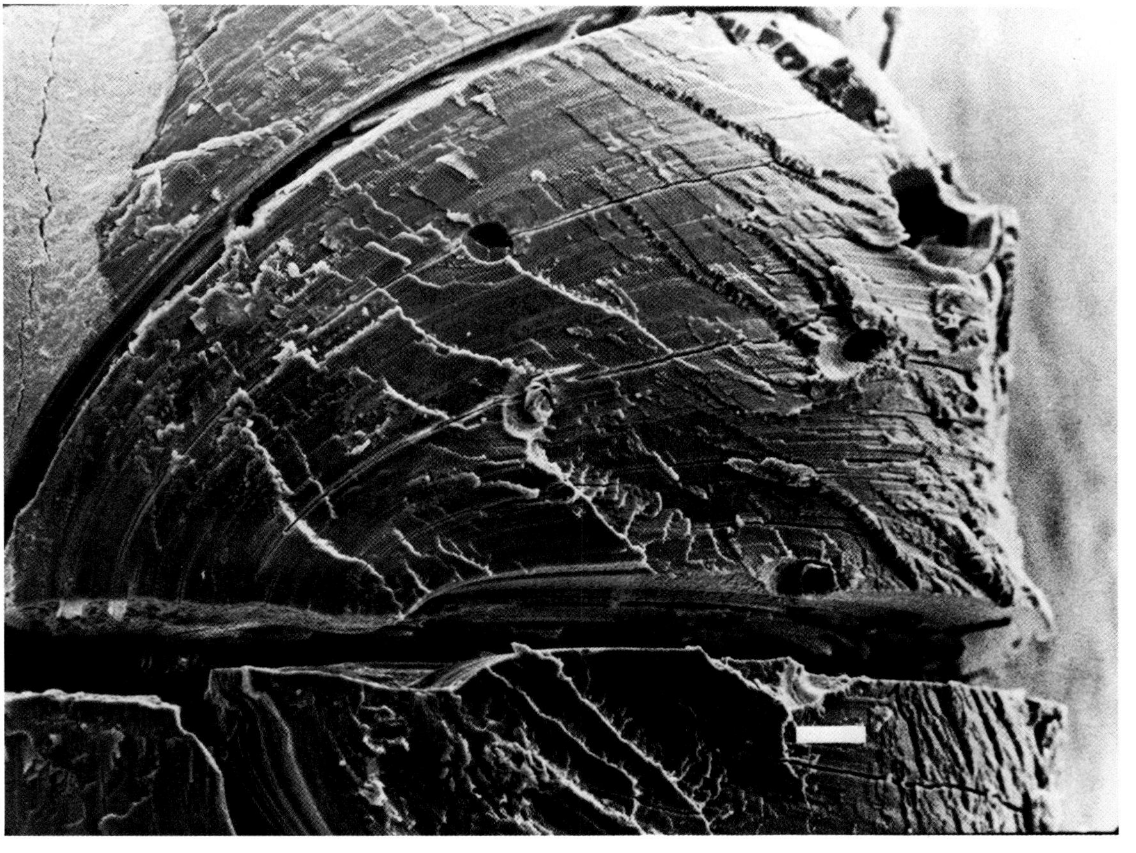

ATLAS Fig. Z. Scanning electron microscope study of modelocked neodymium YAG laser shots on the rabbit lens. Study of the trajectory of a coaxial shot into the rabbit lens cortex: external view. 72 × magnification. The lesion is a well-circumscribed round hole of approximately 90 microns in diameter.

ATLAS Fig. AA. Scanning electron microscope study of modelocked neodymium YAG laser shots on the rabbit lens. Study of the trajectory of a coaxial shot into the rabbit lens cortex: internal view, after sectioning of the lens and removal of the nucleus. 16 × magnification. The entire cortex is perforated by the shot. The total length of the perforation is .225 mm for 2,000 gigawatts. The orifice deep in the cortex measures 70 microns in diameter. The difference in internal and external sizes of the orifice may inpart be due to the photographic technique. There seems to be no transition zone between destroyed and normal cortex.

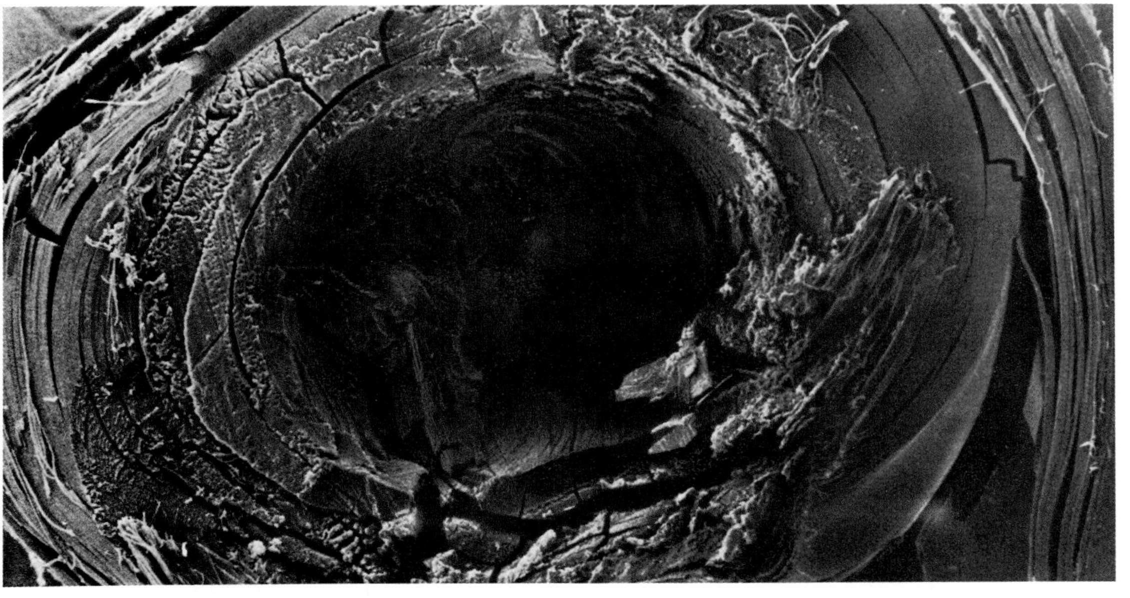

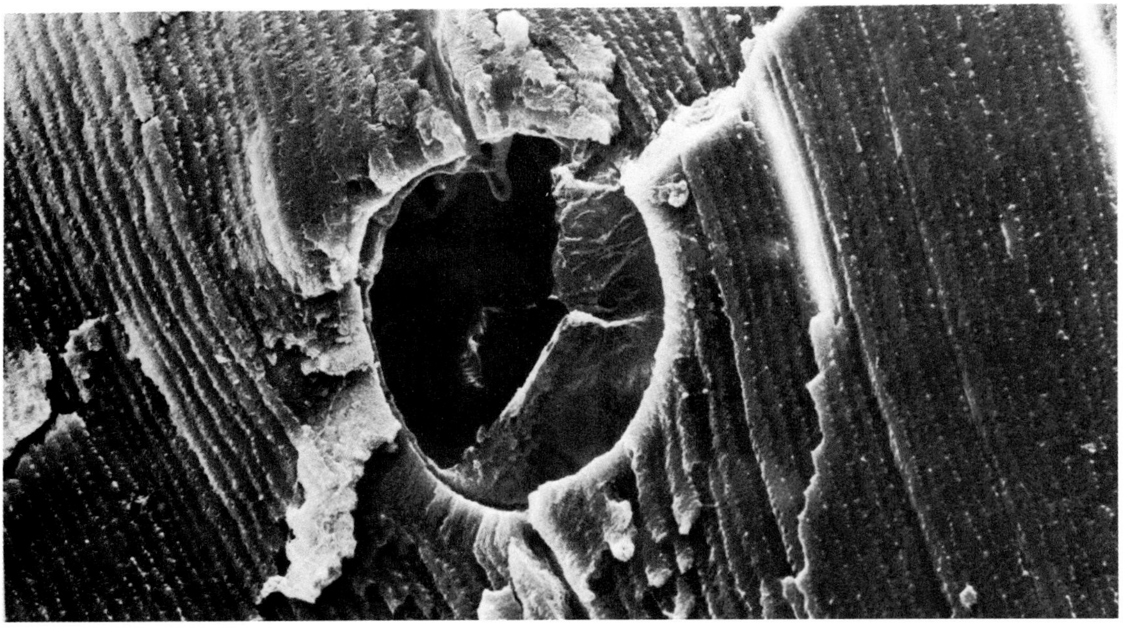

ATLAS Fig. BB. Study at higher magnification of the impact at progressively deeper levels. 500 × magnification. The canal is shown along with the dissociated fibers at the borders of the entry hole. Note the smooth character of the cavity walls.

ATLAS Fig. CC. Study at higher magnification of the impact at progressively deeper levels. 1,200 × magnification. The canal is shown along with the dissociated fibers at the borders of the entry hole.
Note the smooth character of the cavity walls.

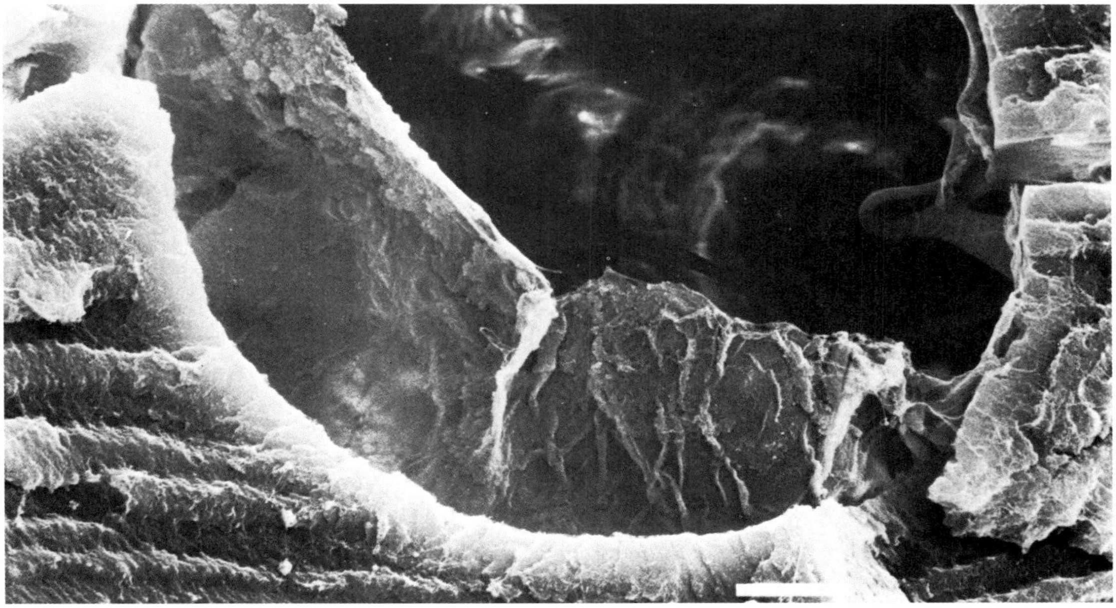

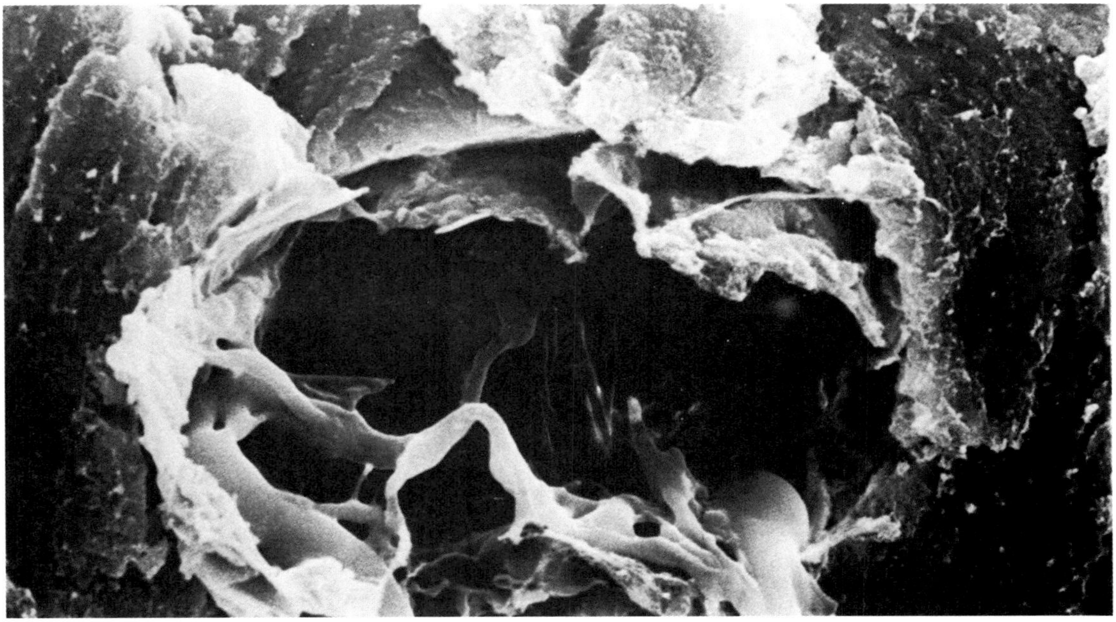

ATLAS Fig. DD. Study at higher magnification of the impact at progressively deeper levels. 1,200 × magnification. The depths of the crater: the explosion zone of a laser shot has a typically round aspect with shredded borders, and shrinkage with loss of normal tissue structure.
The canal is shown along with the dissociated fibers at the borders of the entry hole.

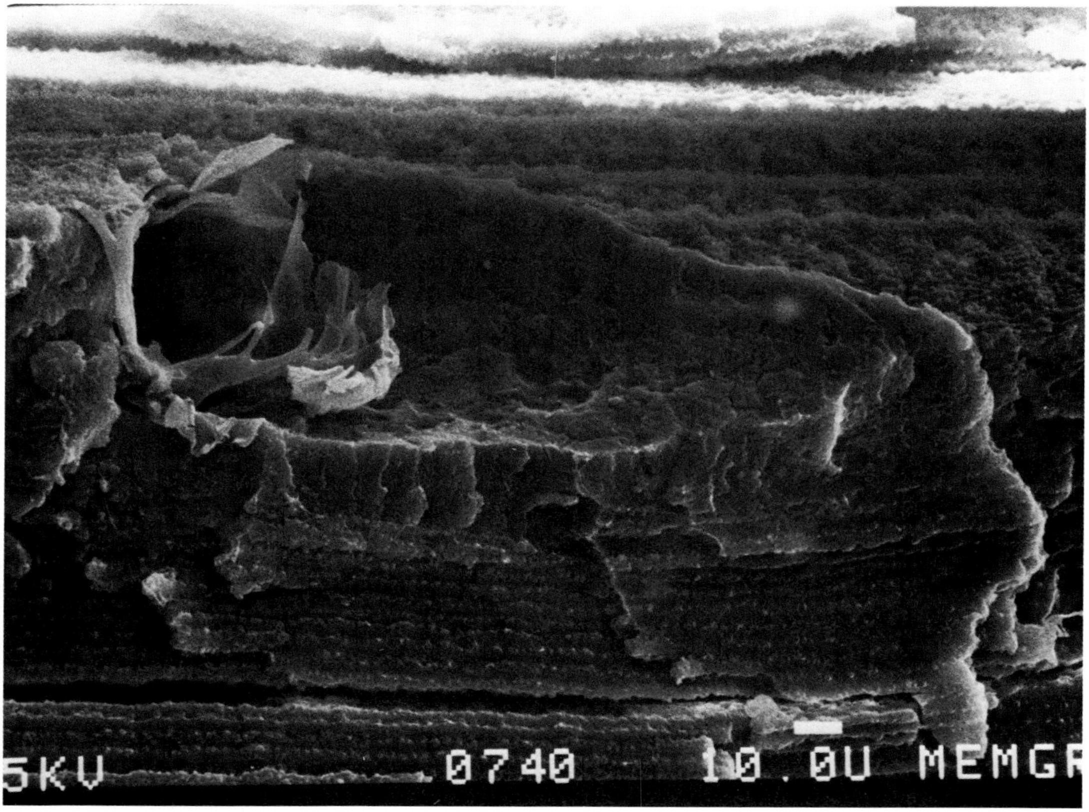

ATLAS Fig. EE. Study of an oblique shot. 500 × magnification. The point of laser focus is to the extreme left of the photo with the reflection of the shock wave travelling antero-laterally.

The closer one comes to the point of focus, the smoother the tunnel walls become. At the other extremity the lens fibers appear more pushed aside than shrunken.

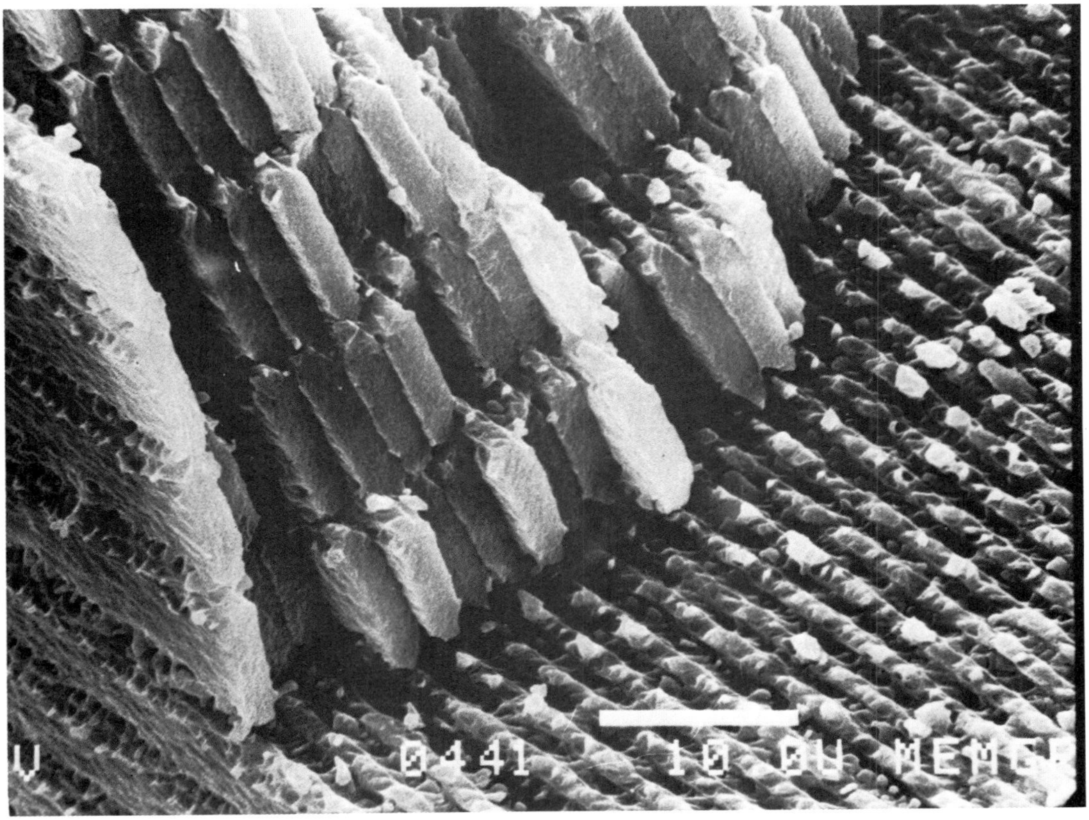

ATLAS Fig. FF. Comparison of fibers bordering the lesion and normal lens fibers. Normal fiber arrangement. 2,000 × magnification. Regular stocking of the fibers is clearly seen. There is no exudate.

ATLAS Fig. GG. Comparison of fibers bordering the lesion and normal lens fibers. Around the shot zone: 1,300 × magnification. Stacking is disrupted in certain zones but, above all, the cortical fibers appear emptied of their contents, presenting a honeycomb appearance. Subcapsular globules of epithelium are found around the edges of the lesion.

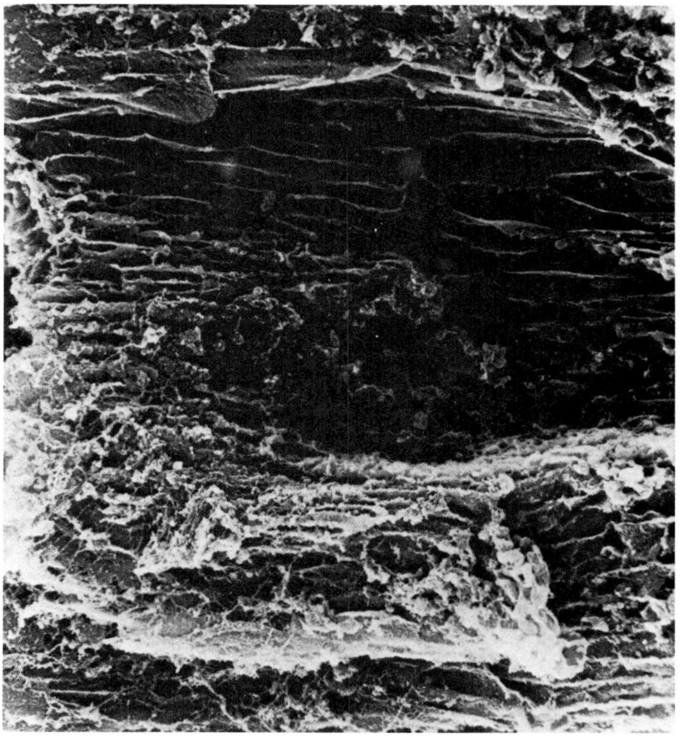

ATLAS Fig. HH. Comparison of fibers bordering the lesion and normal lens fibers. Around the shot zone: 1,300 × magnification. Stocking is disrupted in certain zones but, above all, the cortical fibers appeared emptied of their contents, presenting a honeycomb appearance. Subcapsular globules of epithelium are found around the edges of the lesion.

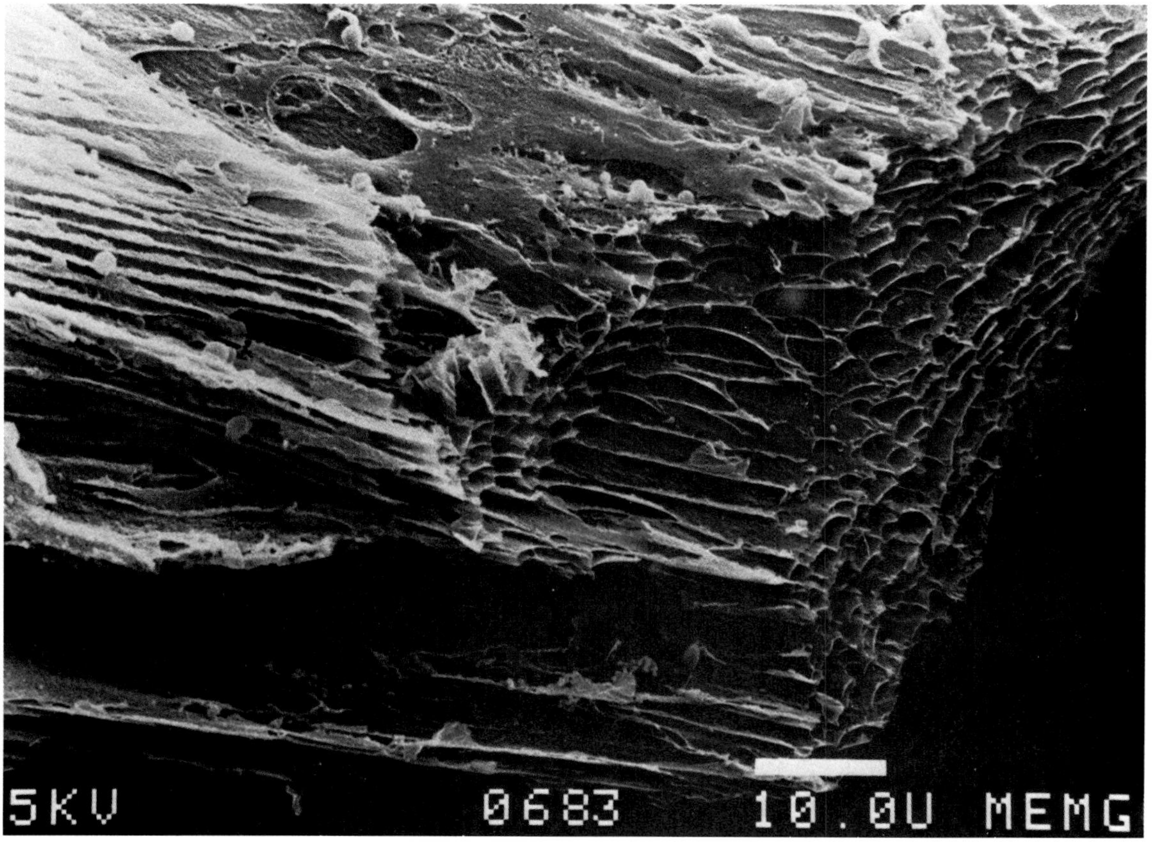

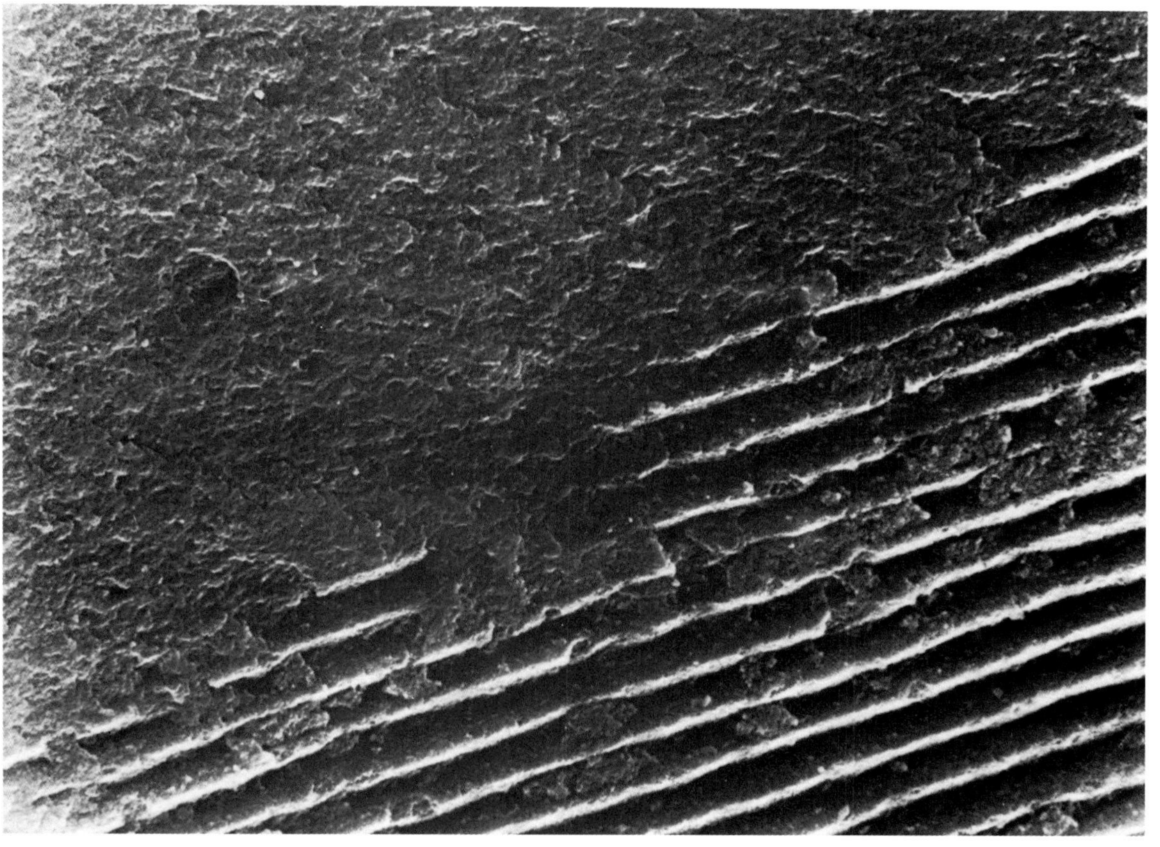

ATLAS Fig. II. Comparison of fibers bordering the lesion and normal lens fibers. Further away: 1,200 × magnification. The fibers are edematous but still maintain their regular structure. They are all covered by an exudate-like material present in greater amounts the closer the shot zone is approached.

ATLAS Fig. JJ. Comparison of fibers bordering the lesion and normal lens fibers. Further away: 1,300 × magnification. The fibers are edematous but still maintain their regular structure. They are all covered by an exudate-like material present in greater amounts the closer the shot zone is approached.

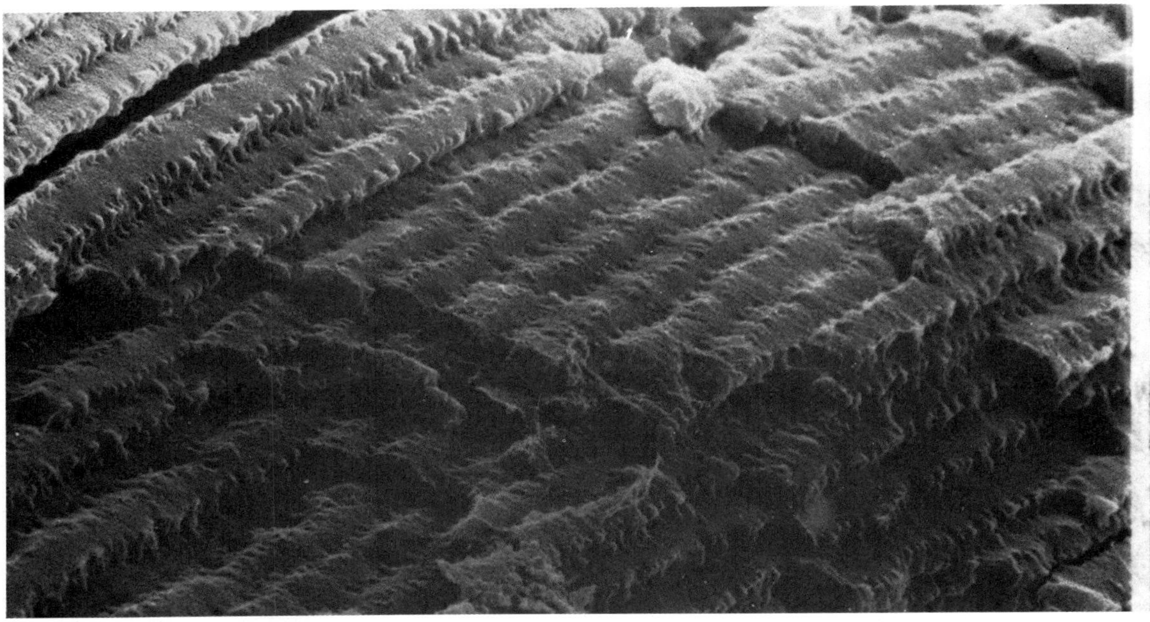

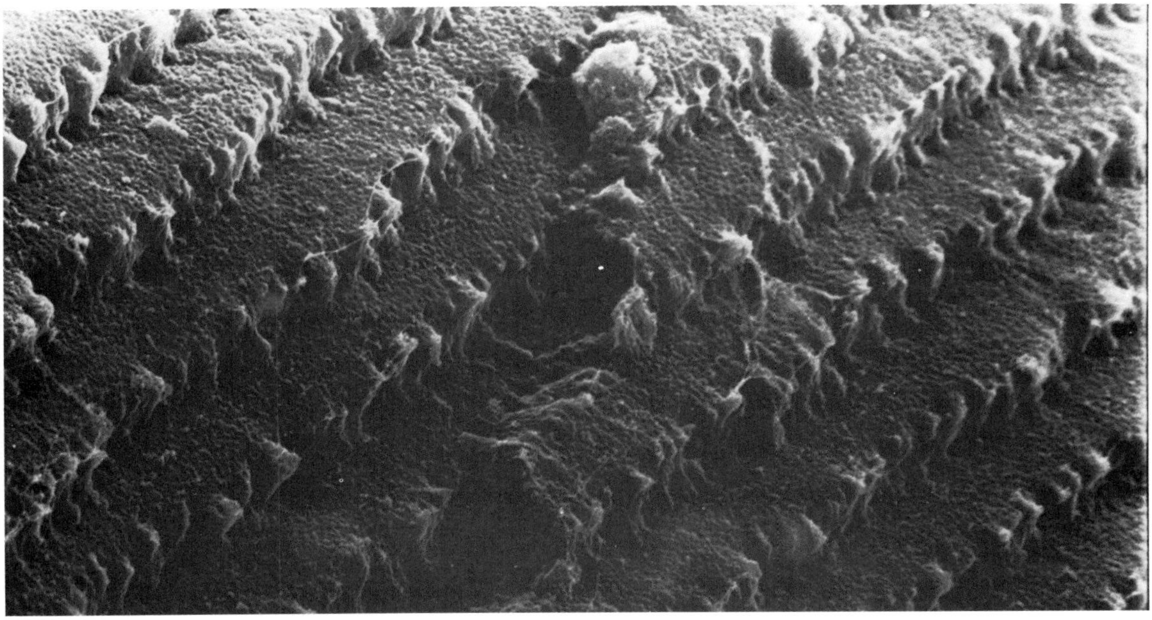

ATLAS Fig. KK. Comparison of fibers bordering the lesion and normal lens fibers. Further away: 3,280 × magnification. The fibers are edematous but still maintain their regular structure. They are all covered by an exudate-like material present in greater amounts the closer the shot zone is approached.

ATLAS Fig. LL. Study of a shot on the anterior lens capsule. Normal aspect of the lens capsule surface: 100 × magnification.

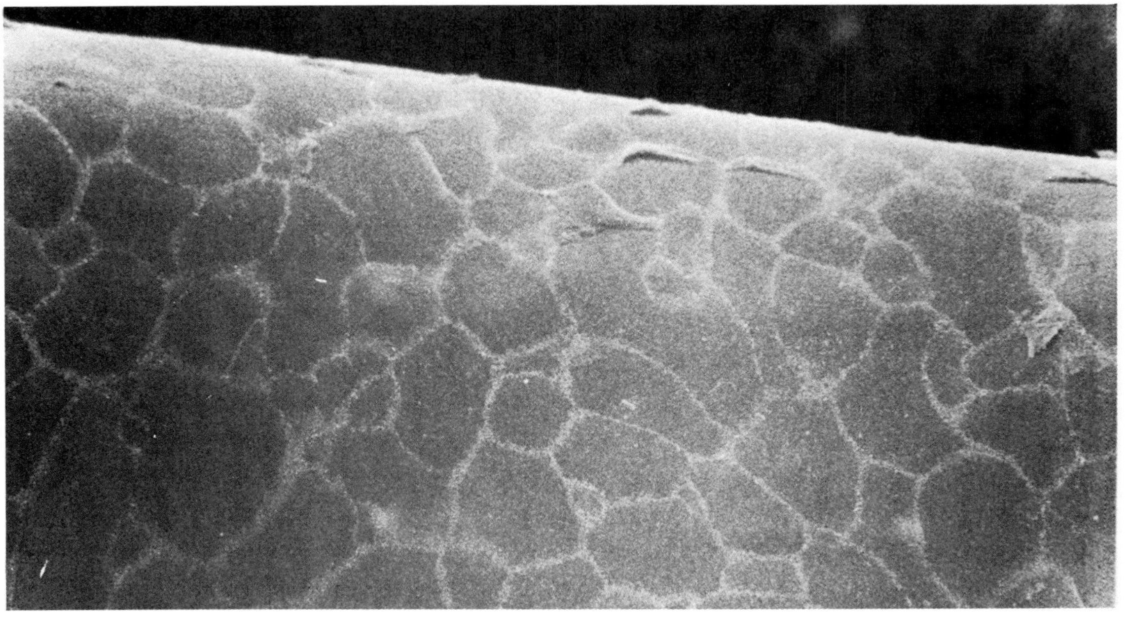

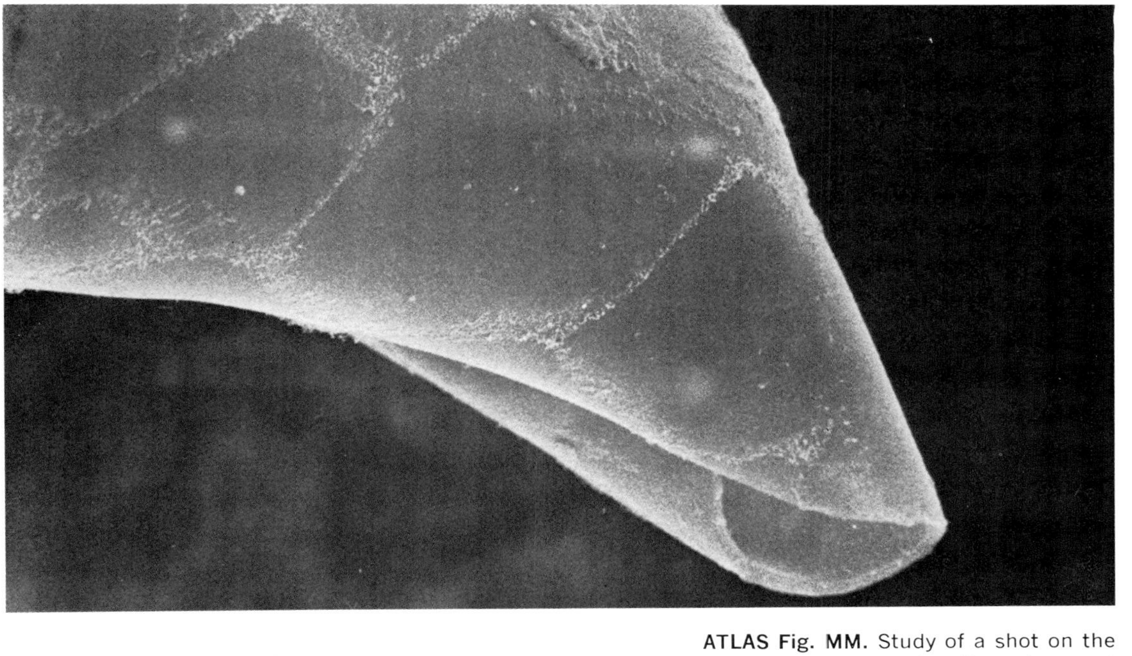

ATLAS Fig. MM. Study of a shot on the anterior lens capsule. Normal aspect of the lens capsule surface: 1000 × magnification.

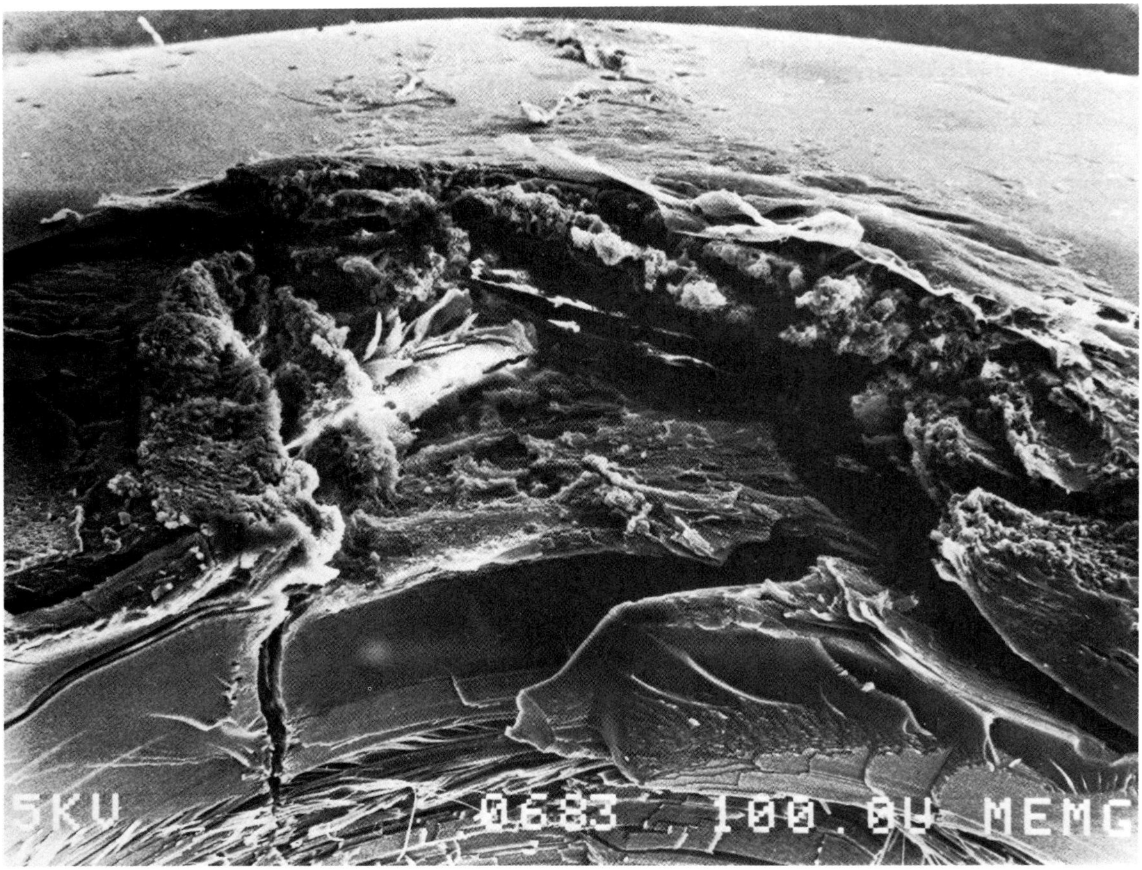

ATLAS Fig. NN. Study of a shot on the anterior lens capsule. Sub-capsular explosion: 100 × magnification. The lens is sectioned at the level of the lesion. The capsule was ruptured by the anterior force of the shock wave. Dissociation and elevation of the cortical fibers are seen.

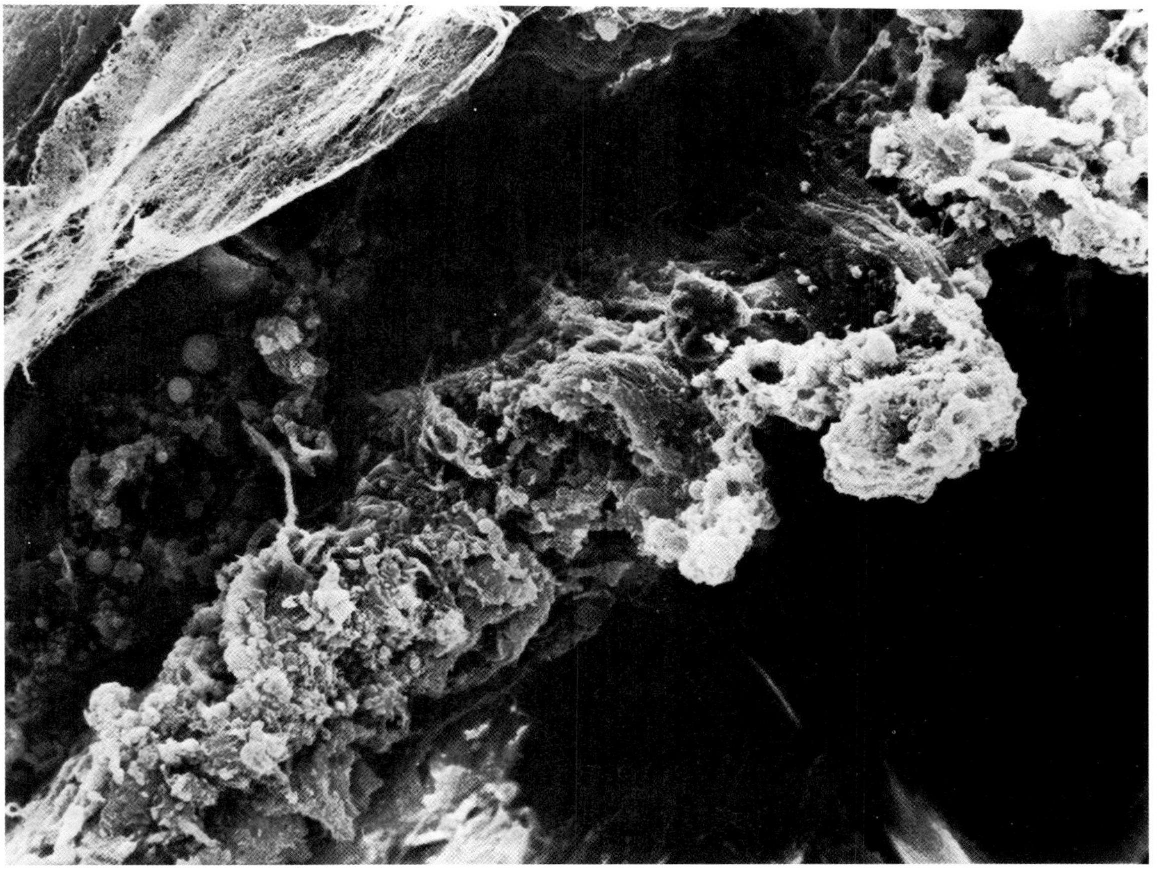

ATLAS Fig. OO. Study of a shot on the anterior lens capsule. At 500 × magnification. The cortical fibers are dissociated and edematous. There are numerous globules of cortex epithelium under the capsule. The capsule is elevated and its edges have a finely-shredded lace-like appearance. This can be compared to the aspect of the normal capsule cut by a blade as seen in 1000 × magnification detail at the extreme left of photo.

ATLAS Fig. PP. Human lens: transmission photography. Anterior capsulotomy and cortex opening; eye removed 18 hours after laser application.

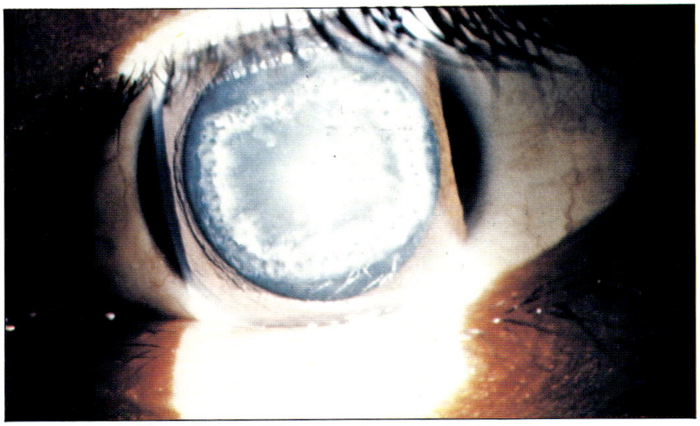

ATLAS Fig. QQ. Human lens: transmission microscopy. Cut section of the anterior capsule.

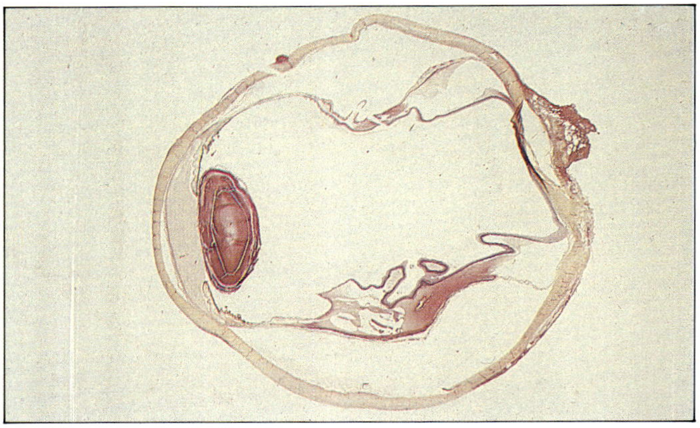

ATLAS Fig. RR. Human lens: transmission microscopy. Erruption of cortex epithelium lens globules, in the anterior chamber.

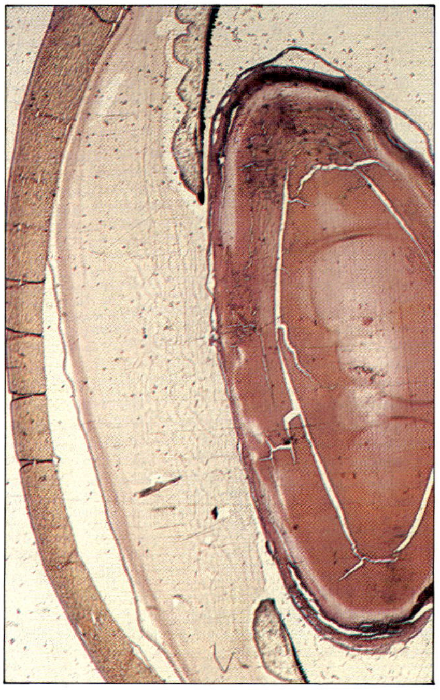

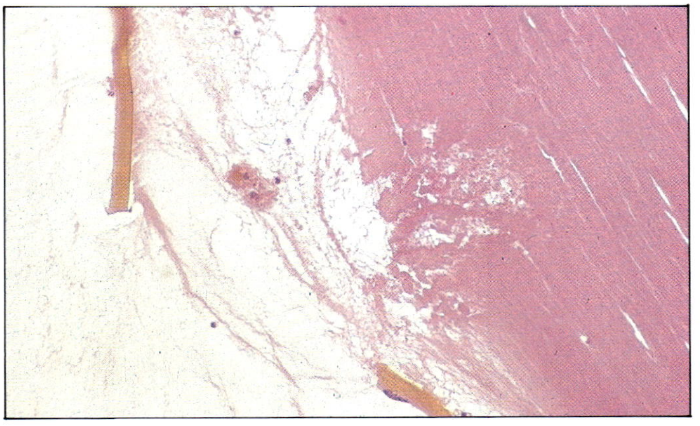

ATLAS Fig. SS. Human lens: transmission microscopy. Liquified lens material in the anterior chamber.

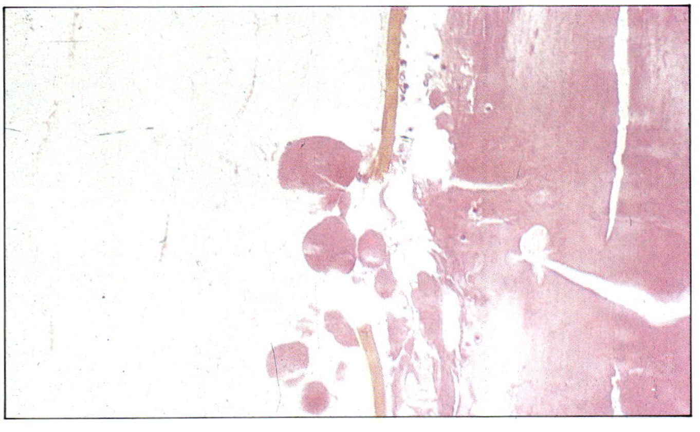

ATLAS Fig. TT. Human lens: transmission microscopy. Normal tension; fine thickness of the capsule makes its rupture wider open than the lens cortex lesion. There was no destruction or burn in the nucleus, the vitreous or on the retina (already detached). Patient age 75 enucleated for painful atrophic eye with retinal detachment.

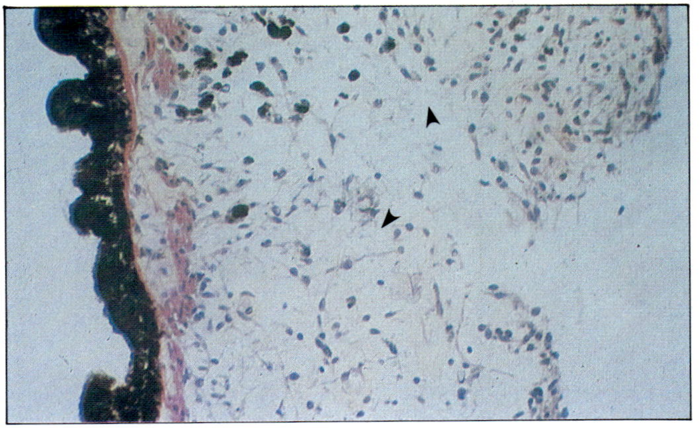

ATLAS Fig. UU. The picosecond monomode modelocked YAG laser-induced lesions on the iris: transmission microscopy. One burst is inefficient and does not perforate the normal iris.

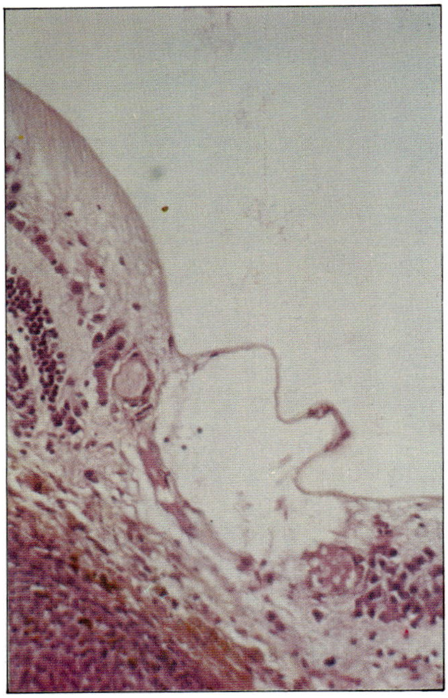

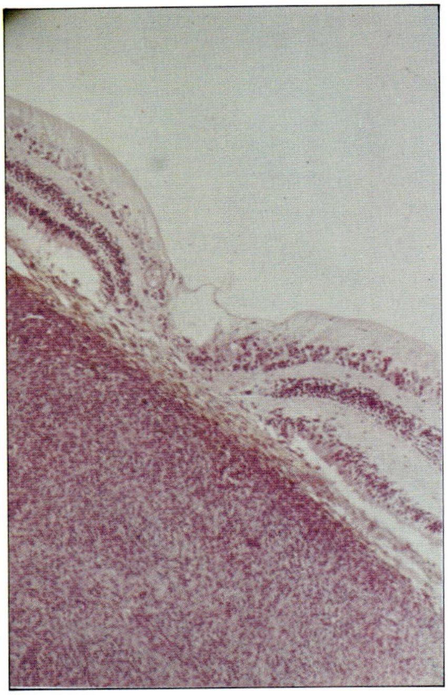

ATLAS Fig. VV. The picosecond mono-mode modelocked YAG laser-induced retinal lesions. Human retina 6 days after laser applications. Output energy 3 to 4 millijoules. Laser focused on the retina.

ATLAS Fig. WW. The picosecond mono-mode modelocked YAG laser-induced retinal lesions. Human retina 6 days after laser applications. Output energy 3 to 4 millijoules. Laser focused on the retina.

ATLAS Fig. XX. The picosecond mono-mode modelocked YAG laser-induced retinal lesions. Picolaser-induced lesions at 6.5 millijoules output energy. Laser focused on the retina. Eye removed on the fourth day.
A. Fluorescein angiography (2nd day); no CME. No leakage around the laser shot which is located on a blood vessel. Hemorrhage pouring in the vitreous.
B, C. Pathology of the retina; Same eye. Removed on the fourth day. Retinal perforation; limited surrounding swelling. Hemorrhage pouring in the vitreous. No lesion on the choroid nor on the sclera.

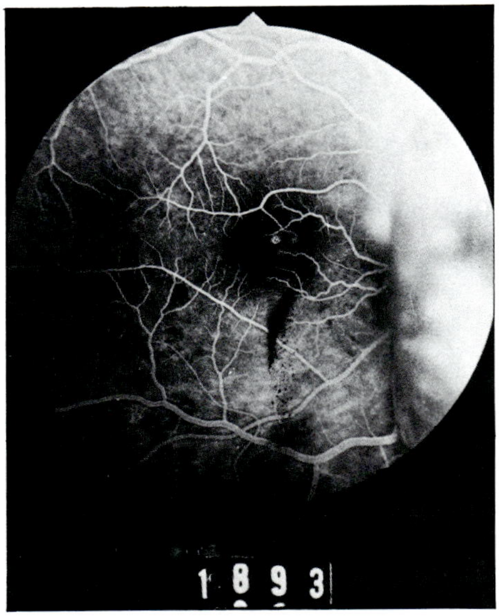

ATLAS Fig. XX (A).

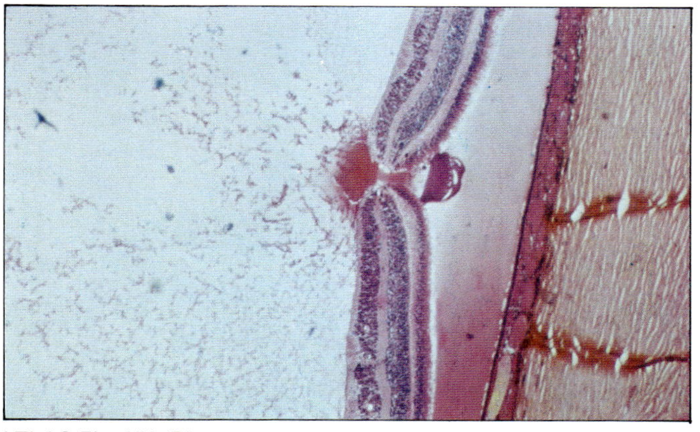
ATLAS Fig. XX (B).

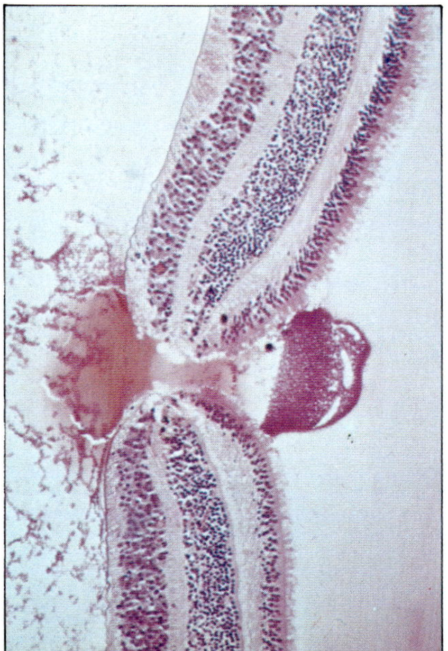
ATLAS Fig. XX (C).

ATLAS Fig. YY. Attempt of trabeculo-puncture of human eye with picosecond mode locked laser, trabeculectomy and trabeculum removed 72 hours later, showing: rupture of the anterior fibers of the trabeculum; cleft in the trabeculum which may be an artifact; no burn, no extensive necrosis, no exudation.

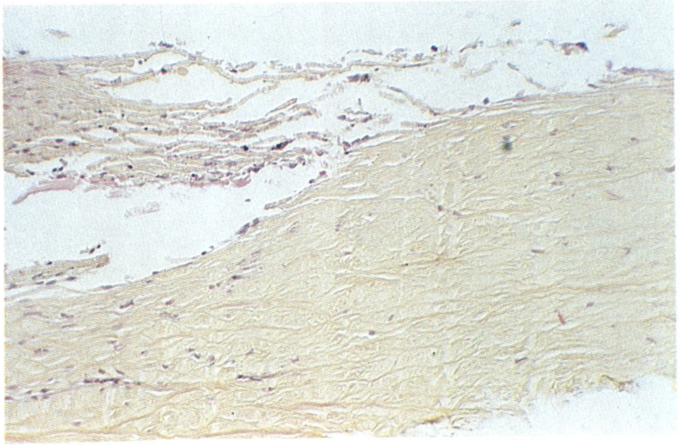

INDEX